SIXTH EDITION

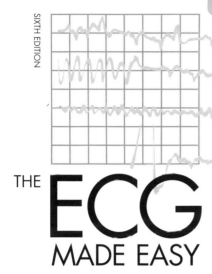

THE
ECG
MADE EASY

Commissioning Editor: Laurence Hunter
Project Development Manager: Lynn Watt and Helius
Project Manager: Nancy Arnott
Designer: Erik Bigland and Helius
Illustrator: Gecko Ltd and Helius
Illustration Manager: Bruce Hogarth

SIXTH EDITION

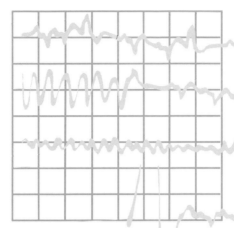

THE ECG
MADE EASY

John R. Hampton DM MA DPhil FRCP FFPM FESC

Emeritus Professor of Cardiology
University of Nottingham
Nottingham
UK

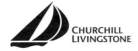

CHURCHILL
LIVINGSTONE

EDINBURGH LONDON NEW YORK OXFORD PHILADELPHIA
ST LOUIS SYDNEY TORONTO 2003

CHURCHILL LIVINGSTONE An imprint of Elsevier Science Limited

First edition 1973
Second edition 1980
Third edition 1986
Fourth edition 1992
Fifth edition 1997
Sixth edition 2003

Standard edition ISBN 0 443 072523
International edition ISBN 0 443 072531

British Library Cataloguing in Publication Data
A catalogue record for this book is available from the British Library

Library of Congress Cataloging in Publication Data
A catalog record for this book is available from the Library of Congress

Note
Medical knowledge is constantly changing. Standard safety precautions must be followed, but as new research and clinical experience broaden our knowledge, changes in treatment and drug therapy may become necessary or appropriate. Readers are advised to check the most current product information provided by the manufacturer of each drug to be administered to verify the recommended dose, the method and duration of administration, and contraindications. It is the responsibility of the practitioner, relying on experience and knowledge of the patient, to determine dosages and the best treatment for each individual patient. Neither the Publisher nor the author assumes any liability for any injury and/or damage to persons or property arising from this publication.

your source for books,
journals and multimedia
in the health sciences

www.elsevierhealth.com

The
publisher's
policy is to use
**paper manufactured
from sustainable forests**

Printed in China

Preface

The ECG Made Easy was first published in 1973, and over a quarter of a million copies of the English language version of the first five editions have been sold. The book has been translated into German, French, Spanish, Italian, Portuguese, Polish, Indonesian and Japanese. The aims of this new edition are the same as before: the book is not intended to be a comprehensive textbook on electrophysiology, nor even of ECG interpretation, but it is designed as an introduction to the ECG for medical students, nurses and paramedics. In addition, it may provide useful revision for those who have forgotten what they learned as students.

There really is no need for the ECG to be daunting: just as most people drive a car without knowing much about engines, and gardeners do not need to be botanists, most people can make full and proper use of the ECG without getting submerged in its complexities. This book encourages the reader to accept that the ECG really is easy to understand, and that its use is just a natural extension of the history and the physical examination.

This is the sixth edition of the book. The text has been changed a little, but the changes to the illustrations are more important. There is a new emphasis on full (12-lead) ECGs, presented in as realistic a way as possible. Examination of a 12-lead ECG gives the best chance of making a diagnosis, and a clinician needs to get into the habit of looking at ECGs presented this way. At the end of the book there is a new section so that you can test yourself and see what you have learned.

The ECG Made Easy should help the student to prepare for examinations, but for the development of clinical competence – and confidence – there is no substitute for reporting on large numbers of clinical records. Two companion texts may help those who have mastered *The ECG Made Easy* and want to progress further. *The ECG in Practice* deals with the relationship between the patient's history and physical signs and the ECG, and with the many variations in the ECG seen in health and disease. *150 ECG Problems* describes 150 clinical cases and gives their full ECGs, in a format that encourages the reader to interpret the record and decide on a course of treatment before looking at the answers.

The title *The ECG Made Easy* was suggested 30 years ago by the late Tony Mitchell, Foundation Professor of Medicine at the University of Nottingham. I am grateful to him and to the many people who have helped to refine the book over the years, and particularly to many students for their constructive criticisms and helpful comments, which have reinforced my belief that the ECG really is easy to understand.

John R. Hampton
Nottingham

Contents

1
What the ECG is about

ECG stands for electrocardiogram, or electrocardiograph. In some countries, the abbreviation used is 'EKG'. Remember:

- By the time you have finished this book, you should be able to say 'The ECG is easy to understand'.
- Most abnormalities of the ECG are amenable to reason.

WHAT TO EXPECT FROM THE ECG

Clinical diagnosis depends mainly on a patient's history, and to a lesser extent on the physical examination. The ECG can provide evidence to support a diagnosis, and in some cases it is crucial for patient management. It is, however, important to see the ECG as a tool, and not as an end in itself.

The ECG is essential for the diagnosis, and therefore management, of abnormal cardiac rhythms. It helps with the diagnosis of the cause of chest pain, and the proper use of thrombolysis in treating myocardial infarction depends upon it. It can help with the diagnosis of the cause of breathlessness.

With practice, interpreting the ECG is a matter of pattern recognition. However, the ECG can be analysed from first principles if a few simple rules and basic facts are remembered. This chapter is about these rules and facts.

THE ELECTRICITY OF THE HEART

The contraction of any muscle is associated with electrical changes called 'depolarization', and these changes can be detected by electrodes attached to the surface of the body. Since all muscular contraction will be detected, the electrical changes associated with contraction of the heart muscle will only be clear if the patient is fully relaxed and no skeletal muscles are contracting.

Although the heart has four chambers, from the electrical point of view it can be thought of as having only two, because the two atria contract together and then the two ventricles contract together.

The wiring diagram of the heart (Fig. 1.1)

The electrical discharge for each cardiac cycle normally starts in a special area of the right atrium called the 'sinoatrial (SA) node'. Depolarization then spreads through the atrial muscle fibres. There is a delay while the depolarization spreads through another special area in the atrium, the 'atrioventricular node' (also called the 'AV

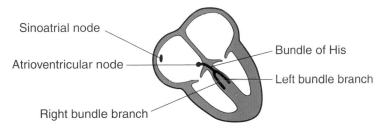

Sinoatrial node

Atrioventricular node

Right bundle branch

Bundle of His

Left bundle branch

Fig. 1.1 The wiring diagram of the heart

node', or sometimes just 'the node'). Thereafter, the electrical discharge travels very rapidly, down specialized conduction tissue: first a single pathway, the 'bundle of His', which then divides in the septum between the ventricles into right and left bundle branches. The left bundle branch itself divides into two. Within the mass of ventricular muscle, conduction spreads somewhat more slowly, through specialized tissue called 'Purkinje fibres'.

The rhythm of the heart

As we shall see later, electrical activation of the heart can sometimes begin in places other than the SA node. The word 'rhythm' is used to refer to the part of the heart which is controlling the activation sequence. The normal heart rhythm, with electrical activation beginning in the SA node, is called 'sinus rhythm'.

THE SHAPE OF THE ECG

The muscle mass of the atria is small compared with that of the ventricles, and the electrical change accompanying the contraction of the atria is therefore small. Contraction of the atria is associated with the ECG wave called 'P'. The ventricular mass is large, and so there is a large deflection of

3

the ECG when the ventricles are depolarized. This is called the 'QRS' complex. The 'T' wave of the ECG is associated with the return of the ventricular mass to its resting electrical state ('repolarization').

The basic shape of the normal ECG is shown in Figure 1.2.

The letters P, Q, R, S and T were selected in the early days of ECG history, and were chosen arbitrarily. The P, Q, R, S and T deflections are all called waves; the Q, R and S waves together make up a complex; and the interval between the S wave and the T wave is called the ST 'segment'.

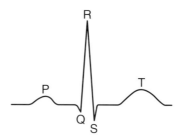

Fig. 1.2 Basic shape of the normal ECG

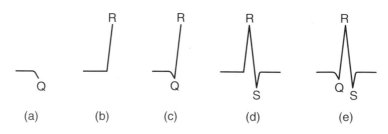

Fig. 1.3 Parts of the QRS complex. (a) Q wave. (b, c) R waves. (d, e) S waves

The different parts of the QRS complex are labelled as shown in Figure 1.3. If the first deflection is downward, it is called a Q wave (Fig. 1.3a). An upward deflection is called an R wave (Fig. 1.3b) – whether it is preceded by a Q wave or not (Fig. 1.3c). Any deflection below the baseline following an R wave is called an S wave (Fig. 1.3d) – whether there has been a preceding Q wave or not (Fig. 1.3e).

Times and speeds

ECG machines record changes in electrical activity by drawing a trace on a moving paper strip. All ECG machines run at a standard rate and use paper with standard-sized squares. Each large square (5 mm) represents 0.2 seconds (s), or 200 milliseconds (ms), so there are five large squares per second, and 300 per minute (min). So an ECG event, such as a QRS complex, occurring once per large square is occurring at a rate of 300/min (Fig. 1.4). The heart rate

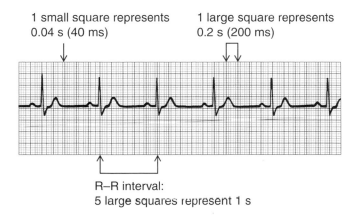

1 small square represents
0.04 s (40 ms)

1 large square represents
0.2 s (200 ms)

R–R interval:
5 large squares represent 1 s

Fig. 1.4 Relationship between the squares on ECG paper and time. Here, there is one QRS complex per second, so the heart rate is 60 beats/min

Table 1.1 Relationship between the number of large squares covered by the R–R interval and the heart rate

R–R interval (large squares)	Heart rate (beats/min)
1	300
2	150
3	100
4	75
5	60
6	50

can be calculated rapidly by remembering the sequence in Table 1.1.

Just as the length of paper between R waves gives the heart rate, so the distance between the different parts of the P–QRS–T complex shows the time taken for conduction of the electrical discharge to spread through the different parts of the heart.

The PR interval is measured from the beginning of the P wave to the beginning of the QRS complex, and is the time taken for excitation to spread from the SA node, through the atrial muscle and the AV node, down the bundle of His and into ventricular muscle.

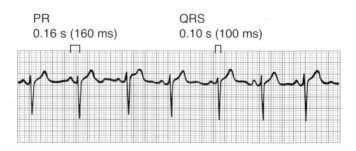

PR
0.16 s (160 ms)

QRS
0.10 s (100 ms)

Fig. 1.5 Duration of the PR interval

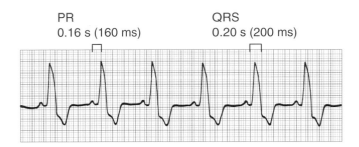

Fig. 1.6 Duration of the QRS complex

The normal PR interval is 0.12–0.2 s (120–200 ms), represented by three to five small squares. Most of the time is taken up by delay in the AV node (Fig. 1.5). If the PR interval is very short, either the atria have been depolarized from close to the AV node, or there is abnormally fast conduction from the atria to the ventricles.

The duration of the QRS complex shows how long excitation takes to spread through the ventricles. The QRS duration is normally 0.12 s (120 ms) (represented by three small squares) or less, but any abnormality of conduction takes longer, and causes widened QRS complexes (Fig. 1.6).

RECORDING AN ECG

The word 'lead' sometimes causes confusion. Sometimes it is used to mean the pieces of wire that connect the patient to the ECG recorder. Properly, a lead is an electrical picture of the heart.

The electrical signal from the heart is detected at the surface of the body through five electrodes, which are joined to the ECG recorder by wires. One electrode is attached to each limb, and one is held by suction to the front of the chest and moved to different positions. Good electrical contact between the electrodes and skin is essential. It may be necessary to shave the chest.

The ECG recorder compares the electrical activity detected in the different electrodes, and the electrical picture so obtained is called a 'lead'. The different comparisons 'look at' the heart from different directions. For example, when the recorder is set to 'lead I' it is comparing the electrical events detected by the electrodes attached to the right and left arms. Each lead gives a different view of the electrical activity of the heart, and so a different ECG pattern. Strictly, each ECG pattern should be called 'lead ...', but often the word 'lead' is omitted.

It is not necessary to remember which electrodes are involved in which leads, but it is essential that the electrodes are properly attached, with the wires labelled 'LA' and 'RA' connected to the left and right arms, respectively, and those labelled 'LL' and 'RL' to the left and right legs, respectively. As we shall see, the ECG is made up of characteristic pictures, and the record as a whole is almost uninterpretable if the electrodes are wrongly attached.

The 12-lead ECG

ECG interpretation is easy if you remember the directions from which the various leads look at the heart. The six 'standard' leads, which are recorded from the electrodes attached to the limbs, can be thought of as looking at the heart in a vertical plane (i.e. from the sides or the feet) (Fig. 1.7).

Leads I, II and VL look at the left lateral surface of the heart, leads III and VF at the inferior surface, and lead VR looks at the right atrium.

The V leads are attached to the chest wall by means of a suction electrode, and recordings are made from six

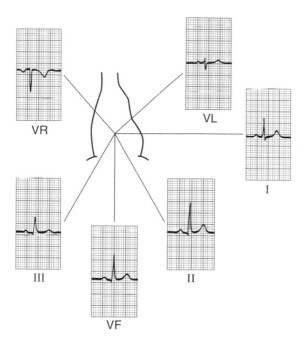

Fig. 1.7 The ECG patterns recorded by the six 'standard' leads

positions, overlying the fourth and fifth rib spaces as shown in Figure 1.8.

The six numbered V leads look at the heart in a horizontal plane, from the front and the left side (Fig. 1.9).

Thus, leads V_1 and V_2 look at the right ventricle, V_3 and V_4 look at the septum between the ventricles and the anterior wall of the left ventricle, and V_5 and V_6 look at the anterior and lateral walls of the left ventricle. As with the limb leads, the chest leads each show a different ECG pattern (Fig. 1.10). In each lead the pattern is characteristic, being similar in different individuals who have normal hearts.

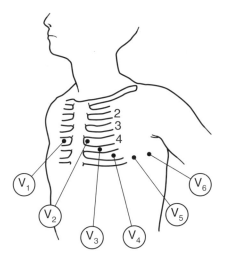

Fig. 1.8 Positioning of the chest V leads. Note that the rib spaces are numbered

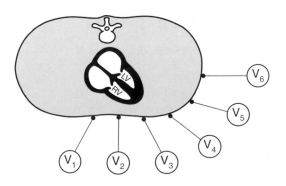

Fig. 1.9 The relationship between the six V leads and the heart

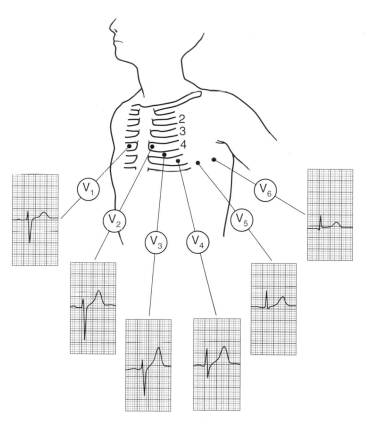

Fig. 1.10 The ECG patterns recorded by the V leads

Calibration

A limited amount of information is provided by the height of the P waves, QRS complexes and T waves, provided the machine is properly calibrated. For example, small complexes may indicate a pericardial effusion, and tall R waves may indicate left ventricular hypertrophy (see Ch. 4). A standard signal of 1 millivolt (mV) should move the stylus

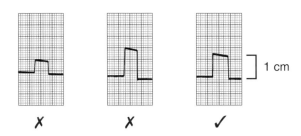

Fig. 1.11 Calibration of the ECG recording

vertically 1 cm (two large squares) (Fig. 1.11), and this 'calibration' signal should be included with every record.

Making a recording
When making a recording:

1. The patient must lie down and relax (to prevent muscle tremor)
2. Connect up the limb electrodes, making certain that they are applied to the correct limb
3. Calibrate the record with the 1 mV signal
4. Record the six standard leads – three or four complexes are sufficient for each
5. Record the six V leads.

THE SHAPE OF THE QRS COMPLEX

We now need to consider why the ECG has a characteristic appearance in each lead.

The QRS complex in the limb leads
The ECG machine is arranged so that when a depolarization wave spreads towards a lead the stylus moves upwards, and when it spreads away from the lead the stylus moves downwards.

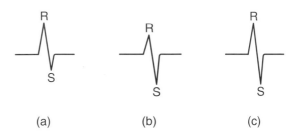

Fig. 1.12 Depolarization and the shape of the QRS complex. Depolarization moving (a) towards the lead, (b) away from the lead and (c) at right angles to the lead

Depolarization spreads through the heart in many directions at once, but the shape of the QRS complex shows the average direction in which the wave of depolarization is spreading through the ventricles (Fig. 1.12).

If the QRS complex is predominantly upward, or positive (i.e. the R wave is greater than the S wave), the depolarization is moving towards that lead (Fig. 1.12a).

If predominantly downward, or negative (S wave greater than R wave), the depolarization is moving away from that lead (Fig. 1.12b).

When the depolarization wave is moving at right angles to the lead, the R and S waves are of equal size (Fig. 1.12c).

Q waves have a special significance, which we shall discuss later.

The cardiac axis

Leads VR and II look at the heart from opposite directions. Seen from the front, the depolarization wave normally spreads through the ventricles from 11 o'clock to 5 o'clock, so the deflections in lead VR are normally mainly downward (negative) and in lead II mainly upward (positive) (Fig. 1.13).

13

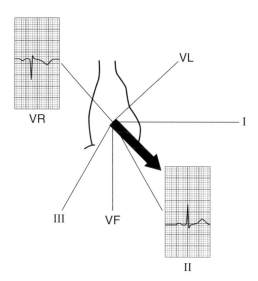

Fig. 1.13 The cardiac axis

The average direction of spread of the depolarization wave through the ventricles as seen from the front is called the 'cardiac axis'. It is useful to decide whether this axis is in a normal direction or not. The direction of the axis can be derived most easily from the QRS complex in leads I, II and III.

A normal 11 o'clock–5 o'clock axis means that the depolarizing wave is spreading towards leads I, II and III and is therefore associated with a predominantly upward deflection in all these leads; the deflection will be greater in lead II than in I or III (Fig. 1.14).

If the right ventricle becomes hypertrophied, the axis will swing towards the right: the deflection in lead I becomes negative (predominantly downward) and the deflection in lead III will become more positive (predominantly upward) (Fig. 1.15). This is called 'right axis deviation'. It is associated mainly with pulmonary conditions that put a strain on the right side of the heart, and with congenital heart disorders.

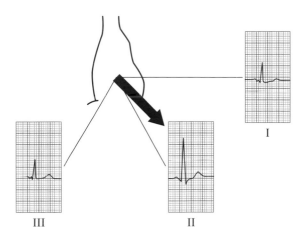

Fig. 1.14 The normal axis

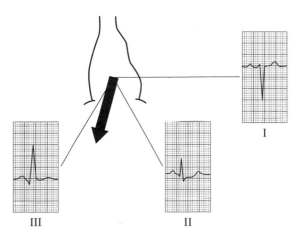

Fig. 1.15 Right axis deviation

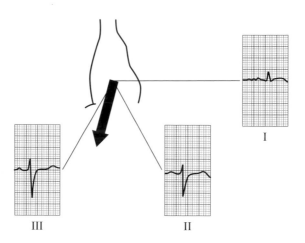

Fig. 1.16 Left axis deviation

When the left ventricle becomes hypertrophied, the axis may swing to the left, so that the QRS complex becomes predominantly negative in lead III (Fig. 1.16). 'Left axis deviation' is not significant until the QRS deflection is also predominantly negative in lead II, and the problem is usually due to a conduction defect rather than to increased bulk of the left ventricular muscle (see Ch. 2).

An alternative explanation of the cardiac axis

Some people find the cardiac axis a difficult concept, and an alternative approach to working it out may be helpful.

The cardiac axis is at right angles (90°) to the lead in which the R and S waves are of equal size (Fig. 1.17).

It is, of course, likely that the axis will not be precisely at right angles to any of the leads, but will be somewhere between two of them. The axis points towards any lead where the R wave is larger than the S wave. It points away from any lead where the S wave is larger than the R wave.

The cardiac axis is sometimes measured in degrees (Fig. 1.18),

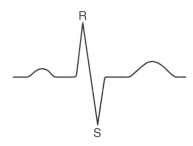

Fig. 1.17 The cardiac axis is at right angles to this lead since the R and S waves are of equal size

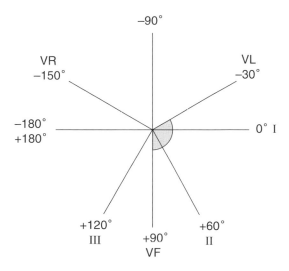

Fig. 1.18 The cardiac axis and lead angle

though this is not clinically particularly useful. Lead I is taken as looking at the heart from 0°; lead II from +60°; lead VF from +90°; and lead III from +120°. Leads VL and VR are said to look from –30° and –150°, respectively.

The normal cardiac axis is in the range –30° to +90°. For example, if in lead II the size of the R wave equals that of the S wave, the axis is at right angles to lead II. In theory, the axis could be at either –30° or +150°. If lead I shows an R wave greater than the S wave, the axis must point towards lead I rather than lead III. Therefore the true axis is at –30° – this is the limit of normality towards what is called the 'left'.

If in lead II the S wave is greater than the R wave, the axis is at an angle of greater than –30°, and left axis deviation is present. Similarly, if the size of the R wave equals that of the S wave in lead I, the axis is at right angles to lead I or at +90°. This is the limit of normality towards the 'right'. If the S wave is greater than the R wave in lead I, the axis is at an angle of greater than +90°, and right axis deviation is present.

Why worry about the cardiac axis?

Right and left axis deviation in themselves are seldom significant – minor degrees occur in long, thin individuals and in short, fat individuals, respectively. However, the presence of axis deviation should alert you to look for other signs of right and left ventricular hypertrophy (see Ch. 4). A change in axis to the right may suggest a pulmonary embolus, and a change to the left indicates a conduction defect.

The QRS complex in the V leads

The shape of the QRS complex in the chest (V) leads is determined by two things:

- The septum between the ventricles is depolarized before the walls of the ventricles, and the depolarization wave spreads across the septum from left to right.

- In the normal heart there is more muscle in the wall of the left ventricle than in that of the right ventricle, and so the left ventricle exerts more influence on the ECG pattern than does the right ventricle.

Leads V_1 and V_2 look at the right ventricle; leads V_3 and V_4 look at the septum; and leads V_5 and V_6 at the left ventricle (see Fig. 1.9).

In a right ventricular lead the deflection is first upwards (R wave) as the septum is depolarized (Fig. 1.19). In a left ventricular lead the opposite pattern is seen: there is a small downward deflection ('septal' Q wave) (Fig. 1.19).

In a right ventricular lead (V_1 and V_2) there is then a downward deflection (S wave) as the main muscle mass is depolarized (Fig. 1.20) – the electrical effects in the bigger left ventricle (in which depolarization is spreading away from a right ventricular lead) outweighing those in the smaller right ventricle (in which depolarization is moving

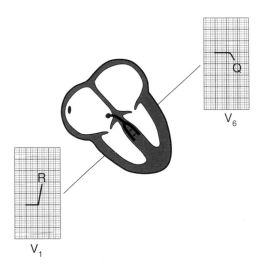

Fig. 1.19 Shape of the QRS complex: first stage

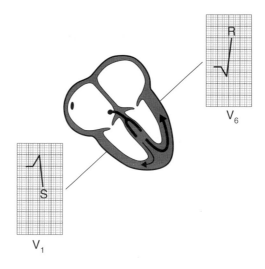

Fig. 1.20 Shape of the QRS complex: second stage

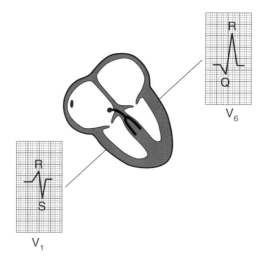

Fig. 1.21 Shape of the QRS complex: third stage

towards a right ventricular lead). In a left ventricular lead there is an upward deflection (R wave) as the ventricular muscle is depolarized (Fig. 1.20).

When the whole of the myocardium is depolarized the ECG returns to baseline (Fig. 1.21).

The QRS complex in the chest leads shows a progression from lead V_1, where it is predominantly downward, to lead V_6, where it is predominantly upward (Fig. 1.22). The

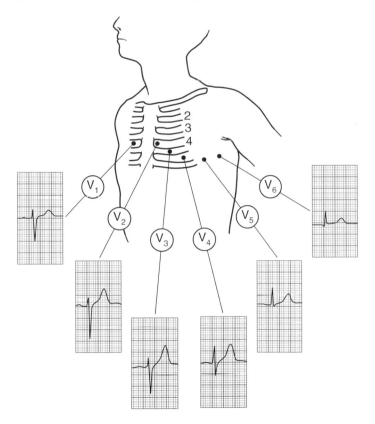

Fig. 1.22 The ECG patterns recorded by the chest leads

'transition point', where the R and S waves are equal, indicates the position of the interventricular septum.

Why worry about the transition point?

If the right ventricle is enlarged, and occupies more of the precordium than is normal, the transition point will move from its normal position of leads V_3/V_4 to leads V_4/V_5 or sometimes leads V_5/V_6. Seen from below, the heart can be thought of as having rotated in a clockwise direction. 'Clockwise rotation' in the ECG is characteristic of chronic lung disease.

HOW TO REPORT AN ECG

You now know enough about the ECG to understand the basis of a report. This should take the form of a description, followed by an interpretation.

The description should always be given in the same sequence:

1. Rhythm
2. Conduction intervals
3. Cardiac axis
4. A description of the QRS complexes
5. A description of the ST segments and T waves.

Reporting a series of totally normal findings is possibly pedantic, and in real life is frequently not done. However, you must think about all the findings every time you interpret an ECG.

ECG INTERPRETATION

The interpretation indicates whether the record is normal or abnormal: if abnormal, the underlying pathology needs to be identified. Examples of 12-lead ECGs are shown in Figures 1.23 and 1.24.

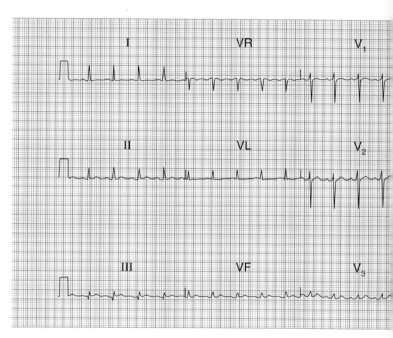

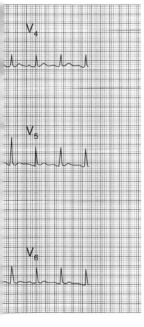

Fig. 1.23 12-lead ECG: example 1

Description
- Sinus rhythm, rate 110/min
- Normal PR interval (140 ms)
- Normal QRS duration (120 ms)
- Normal cardiac axis
- Normal QRS complexes
- Normal T waves (an inverted T wave in lead VR is normal)

Interpretation
- Normal ECG

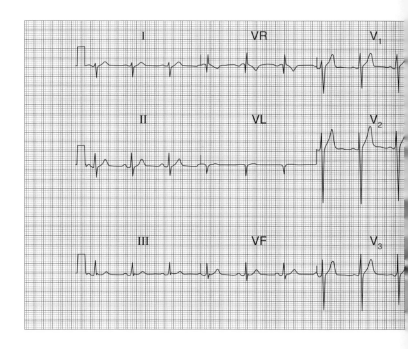

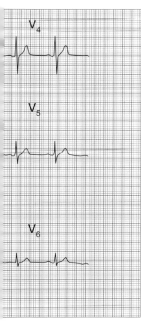

Fig. 1.24 12-lead ECG: example 2

Description
- Sinus rhythm, rate 75/min
- PR interval 200 ms
- QRS duration 120 ms
- Right axis deviation (prominent S wave in lead I)
- Normal QRS complexes
- Normal ST segments and T waves

Interpretation
- Normal ECG – apart from right axis deviation, which could be normal in a tall thin person.

    Unfortunately, there are a lot of minor variations in ECGs which are consistent with perfectly normal hearts. Recognizing the limits of normality is one of the main difficulties of ECG interpretation

THINGS TO REMEMBER

1. The ECG results from electrical changes associated with activation first of the atria and then of the ventricles.
2. Atrial activation causes the P wave.
3. Ventricular activation causes the QRS complex. If the first deflection is downward it is a Q wave. Any upward deflection is an R wave. A downward deflection after an R wave is an S wave.

4. When the depolarization wave spreads towards a lead, the deflection is predominantly upward. When the wave spreads away from a lead, the deflection is predominantly downward.
5. The six limb leads (I, II, III, VR, VL and VF) look at the heart from the sides and the feet in a vertical plane.
6. The cardiac axis is the average direction of spread of depolarization as seen from the front, and is estimated from leads I, II and III.
7. The chest or V leads look at the heart from the front and the left side in a horizontal plane. Lead V_1 is positioned over the right ventricle, and lead V_6 over the left ventricle.
8. The septum is depolarized from the left side to the right.
9. In a normal heart the left ventricle exerts more influence on the ECG than the right ventricle.

2
Conduction and its problems

We have already seen that electrical activation normally
begins in the sinoatrial (SA) node, and that a wave of
depolarization spreads outwards through the atrial muscle
to the atrioventricular (AV) node, and thence down the His
bundle and its branches to the ventricles. The conduction of
this wave front can be delayed or blocked at any point.
However:

- Conduction problems are simple to analyse provided you
  keep the wiring diagram of the heart constantly in mind
  (Fig. 2.1).

We can think of conduction problems in the order
in which the depolarization wave normally spreads: SA
node → AV node → His bundle → bundle branches.

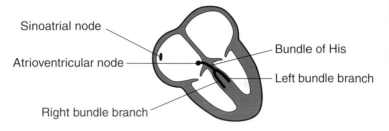

Fig. 2.1 **The wiring diagram of the heart**

Remember in all that follows that we are assuming depolarization begins in the normal way in the SA node.

The rhythm of the heart is best interpreted from whichever ECG lead shows the P wave most clearly. This is usually, but not always, lead II or lead V_1. You can assume that all the 'rhythm strips' in this book were recorded from one of these leads.

CONDUCTION PROBLEMS IN THE AV NODE AND HIS BUNDLE

The time taken for the spread of depolarization from the SA node to the ventricular muscle is shown by the PR interval (see Ch. 1), and is not normally greater than 0.2 s (one large square). ECG events are usually timed in milliseconds rather than seconds, so the limit of the PR interval is 200 ms. Interference with the conduction process causes the ECG phenomenon called 'heart block'.

First degree heart block

If each wave of depolarization that originates in the SA node is conducted to the ventricles, but there is delay somewhere along the conduction pathway, then the PR interval is prolonged. This is called 'first degree heart block' (Fig. 2.2).

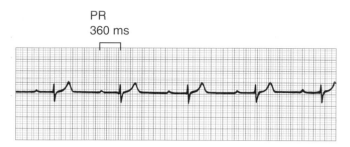

Fig. 2.2 First degree block

Note
- One P wave per QRS complex
- PR interval 360 ms

First degree heart block is not in itself important, but it may be a sign of coronary artery disease, acute rheumatic carditis, digoxin toxicity or electrolyte disturbances.

Second degree heart block

Sometimes excitation completely fails to pass through the AV node or the bundle of His. When this occurs *intermittently*, 'second degree heart block' is said to exist. There are three variations of this:

1. Most beats are conducted with a constant PR interval, but occasionally there is an atrial contraction without a subsequent ventricular contraction. This is called the 'Mobitz type 2' phenomenon (Fig. 2.3).
2. There may be progressive lengthening of the PR interval and then failure of conduction of an atrial beat, followed by a conducted beat with a shorter PR interval and then a repetition of this cycle. This is the 'Wenckebach' phenomenon (Fig. 2.4).
3. There may be alternate conducted and non-conducted atrial beats (or one conducted atrial beat and then two

31

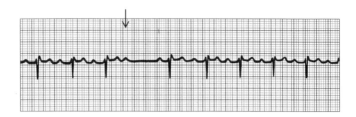

Fig. 2.3 Second degree heart block (Mobitz type 2)

Note
- PR interval of the conducted beats is constant
- One P wave is not followed by a QRS complex, and here second degree block is occurring

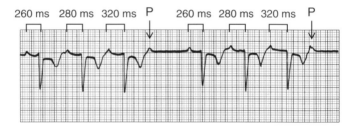

Fig. 2.4 Second degree heart block (Wenckebach type)

Note
- Progressive lengthening of PR interval
- One non-conducted beat
- Next conducted beat has a shorter PR interval than the preceding conducted beat

non-conducted beats), giving twice (or three times) as many P waves as QRS complexes. This is called '2:1' ('two to one') (or '3:1' ('three to one')) conduction (Fig. 2.5).

It is important to remember that, as with any other rhythm, a P wave may only show itself as a distortion of a T wave (Fig. 2.6).

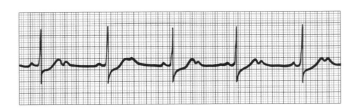

Fig. 2.5 Second degree heart block (2:1 type)

Note
- Two P waves per QRS complex
- Normal, and constant, PR interval in the conducted beats

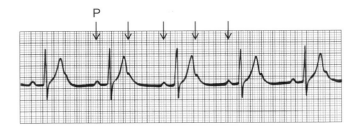

Fig. 2.6 Second degree heart block (2:1 type)

Note
- P wave in the T wave can be identified because of its regularity

The underlying causes of second degree heart block are the same as those of first degree block. The Wenckebach phenomenon is usually benign, but Mobitz type 2 block and 2:1 block may herald 'complete,' or 'third degree', heart block.

Third degree heart block
Complete heart block (third degree block) is said to occur when atrial contraction is normal but no beats are conducted to the ventricles (Fig. 2.7). When this occurs the

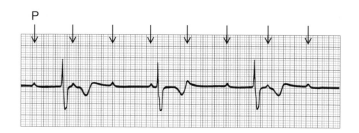

Fig. 2.7 Third degree block

Note
- P wave rate 90/min
- QRS complex rate 36/min
- No relationship between P waves and QRS complexes
- Abnormally-shaped QRS complexes because of abnormal spread of depolarization from a ventricular focus

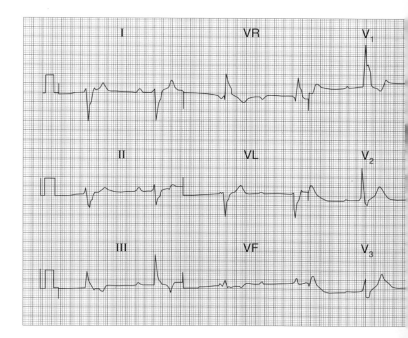

ventricles are excited by a slow 'escape mechanism' (see Ch. 3), from a depolarizing focus within the ventricular muscle.

Complete block is not always immediately obvious in a 12-lead ECG, where there may be only a few QRS complexes per lead (e.g. see Fig. 2.8). You have to look at the PR interval in all the leads.

Complete heart block may occur as an acute phenomenon in patients with myocardial infarction (when it is usually transient) or it may be a chronic state, usually due to fibrosis around the bundle of His. It may also be caused by the block of both bundle branches.

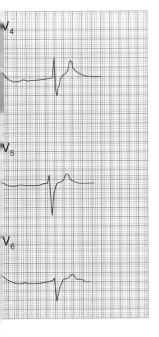

Fig. 2.8 Complete heart block

Note
- Sinus rhythm, but no P waves are conducted
- Right axis deviation
- Broad QRS complexes (duration 160 ms)
- Right bundle branch block pattern
- The cause of the block could not be determined, though in most patients it results from fibrosis of the bundle of His

CONDUCTION PROBLEMS IN THE RIGHT AND LEFT BUNDLE BRANCHES – BUNDLE BRANCH BLOCK

If the depolarization wave reaches the interventricular septum normally, the interval between the beginning of the P wave and the first deflection in the QRS complex (the PR interval) will be normal. However, if there is abnormal conduction through either the right or left bundle branches ('bundle branch block') there will be a delay in the depolarization of part of the ventricular muscle. The extra time taken for depolarization of the whole of the ventricular muscle causes widening of the QRS complex.

In the normal heart, the time taken for the depolarization wave to spread from the interventricular septum to the furthest part of the ventricles is less than 120 ms, represented by three small squares of ECG paper. If the QRS duration is greater than 120 ms, then conduction within the ventricles must have occurred by an abnormal and therefore slow pathway.

Although a wide QRS complex can indicate bundle branch block, widening also occurs if depolarization begins within the ventricular muscle itself (see Ch. 3). Remember that in sinus rhythm with bundle branch block, normal P waves are present with a constant PR interval. We shall see that this is not the case with rhythms beginning in the ventricles.

Block of both bundle branches has the same effect as block of the His bundle, and causes complete (third degree) heart block.

Right bundle branch block (RBBB) often indicates problems in the right side of the heart, but RBBB patterns with a QRS complex of normal duration are quite common in healthy people.

Left bundle branch block (LBBB) is always an indication of heart disease, usually of the left side. It is important to recognize that bundle branch block is present, because

LBBB prevents any further interpretation of the cardiogram, and RBBB can make interpretation difficult.

The mechanism underlying the ECG patterns of RBBB and LBBB can be worked out from first principles. Remember (see Ch. 1):

- The septum is normally depolarized from left to right.
- The left ventricle, having the greater muscle mass, exerts more influence on the ECG than does the right ventricle.
- Excitation spreading towards a lead causes an upward deflection within the ECG.

Right bundle branch block

No conduction occurs down the right bundle branch, but the septum is depolarized from the left side as usual, causing an R wave in a right ventricular lead (V_1) and a small Q wave in a left ventricular lead (V_6) (Fig. 2.9).

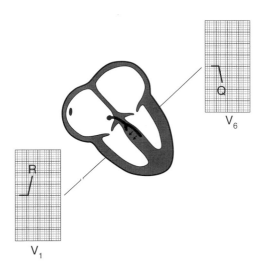

Fig. 2.9 Conduction in right bundle branch block: first stage

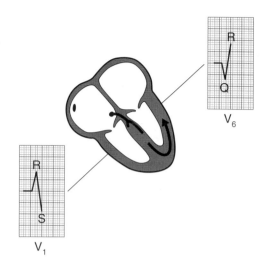

Fig. 2.10 Conduction in right bundle branch block: second stage

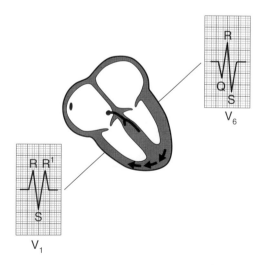

Fig. 2.11 Conduction in right bundle branch block: third stage

Excitation then spreads to the left ventricle, causing an S wave in lead V_1 and an R wave in lead V_6 (Fig. 2.10).

It takes longer than in a normal heart for excitation to reach the right ventricle because of the failure of the normal conducting pathway. The right ventricle therefore depolarizes after the left. This causes a second R wave (R^1) in lead V_1, and a wide and deep S wave in lead V_6 (Fig. 2.11).

An 'RSR^1' pattern, but with a QRS complex of normal width (less than 120 ms), is sometimes called 'partial right bundle branch block'. It is seldom of significance, and can be considered to be a normal variant.

Left bundle branch block

If conduction down the left bundle branch fails, the septum becomes depolarized from right to left, causing a small Q wave in lead V_1, and an R wave in lead V_6 (Fig. 2.12).

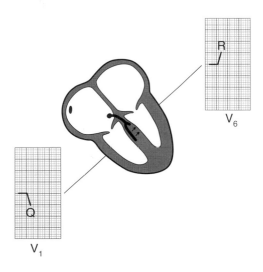

Fig. 2.12 Conduction in left bundle branch block: first stage

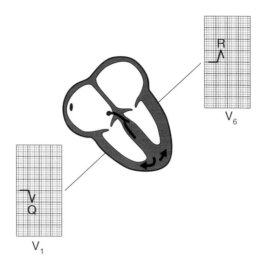

Fig. 2.13 Conduction in left bundle branch block: second stage

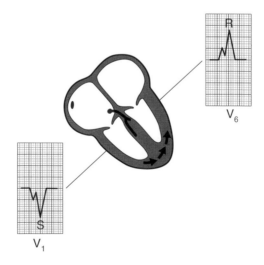

Fig. 2.14 Conduction in left bundle branch block: third stage

The right ventricle is depolarized before the left, so despite the smaller muscle mass there is an R wave in lead V_1 and an S wave (often appearing only as a notch) in lead V_6 (Fig. 2.13).

Subsequent depolarization of the left ventricle causes an S wave in lead V_1 and another R wave in lead V_6 (Fig. 2.14).

LBBB is associated with T wave inversion in the lateral leads (I, V_2 and V_5–V_6).

What to remember

RBBB is best seen in lead V_1 where there is an RSR^1 pattern (Fig. 2.15).

LBBB is best seen in lead V_6, where there is a broad complex with a notched top, which resembles the letter 'M' and is thus known as an 'M' pattern (Fig. 2.16). The complete picture, with a 'W' pattern in lead V_1, is often not fully developed.

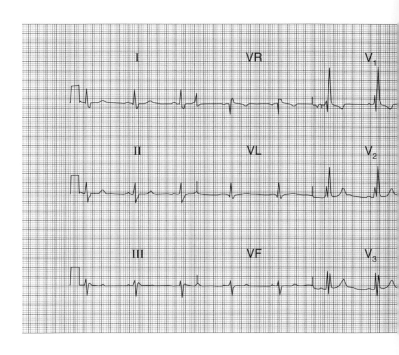

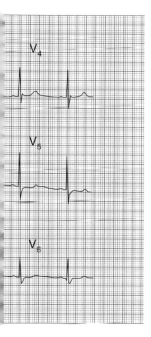

Fig. 2.15 Sinus rhythm with RBBB

Note
- Sinus rhythm, rate 75/min
- Normal PR interval
- Normal cardiac axis
- Wide QRS complexes (160 ms)
- RSR[1] pattern in lead V_1 and deep, wide S waves in lead V_6
- Normal ST segments and T waves

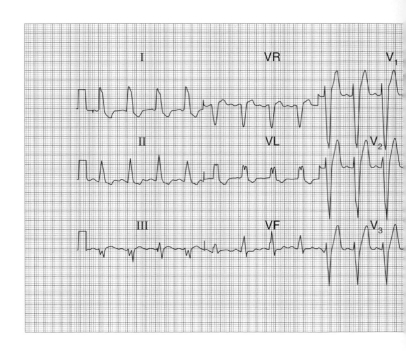

CONDUCTION PROBLEMS IN THE DISTAL PARTS OF THE LEFT BUNDLE BRANCH

At this point it is worth considering in a little more detail the anatomy of the branches of the His bundle. The right bundle branch has no main divisions but the left bundle branch has two – the anterior and posterior 'fascicles'. The depolarization wave therefore spreads into the ventricles by three pathways (Fig. 2.17).

The cardiac axis (see Ch. 1) depends on the average direction of depolarization of the ventricles. Since the left ventricle contains more muscle than the right, it has more influence on the cardiac axis (Fig. 2.18).

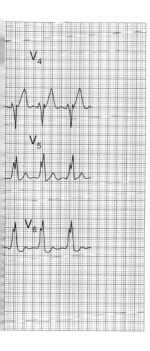

Fig. 2.16 Sinus rhythm with LBBB

Note

- Sinus rhythm, rate 100/min
- Normal PR interval
- Normal cardiac axis
- Wide QRS complexes (160 ms)
- M pattern in the QRS complexes, best seen in leads I, VL, V_5, V_6
- Inverted T waves in leads I, II, VL

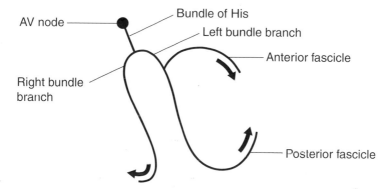

Fig. 2.17 The three pathways of the depolarization wave

If the anterior fascicle of the left bundle branch fails to conduct, the left ventricle has to be depolarized through the posterior fascicle and so the cardiac axis rotates upwards (Fig. 2.19).

Left axis deviation is therefore due to left anterior fascicular block, or 'left anterior hemiblock' (Fig. 2.20).

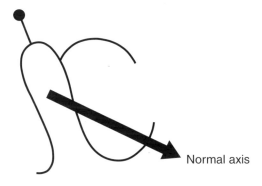

Normal axis

Fig. 2.18 Effect of normal conduction on the cardiac axis

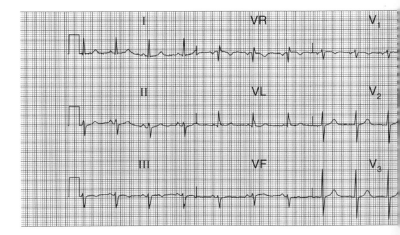

The posterior fascicle of the left bundle is not often selectively blocked, but if this does occur the ECG shows right axis deviation.

When the right bundle branch is blocked, the cardiac axis usually remains normal, because there is normal depolarization of the left ventricle with its large muscle mass (Fig. 2.21).

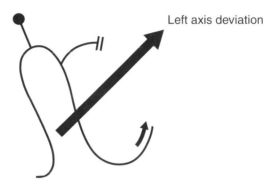

Left axis deviation

Fig. 2.19 Effect of left anterior fascicular block on the cardiac axis

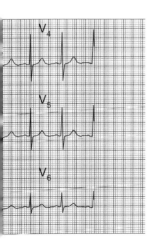

Fig. 2.20 Sinus rhythm with left axis deviation (otherwise normal)

Note
- Sinus rhythm, rate 80/min
- Left axis deviation: QRS complex upright in lead I, but downward (dominant S wave) in leads II and III
- Normal QRS complexes, ST segments and T waves

However, if both the right bundle branch and the left anterior fascicle are blocked, the ECG shows right bundle branch block and left axis deviation (LAD) (Fig. 2.22). This is sometimes called 'bifascicular block', and this particular

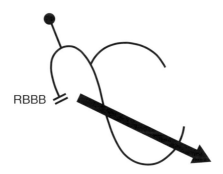

Fig. 2.21 Effect of RBBB on the cardiac axis

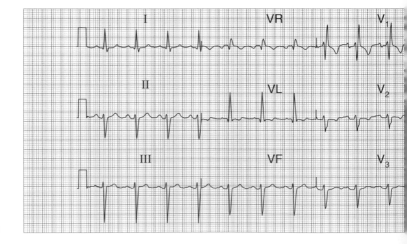

ECG pattern obviously indicates widespread damage to the conducting system (Fig. 2.23).

If the right bundle branch and both fascicles of the left bundle branch are blocked, complete heart block occurs just as if the main His bundle had failed to conduct.

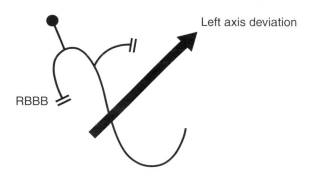

Fig. 2.22 Effect of RBBB and left anterior hemiblock on the cardiac axis

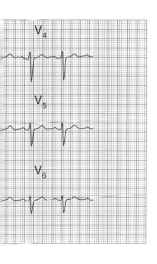

Fig. 2.23 Bifascicular block

Note

- Sinus rhythm, rate 90/min
- Left axis deviation (dominant S wave in leads II and III)
- RBBB (RSR pattern in lead V_1, and deep wide S wave in lead V_6)

WHAT TO DO

Always remember that it is the patient who should be treated, not the ECG. Relief of symptoms always comes first. However, some general points can be made about the action that might be taken if the ECG shows conduction abnormalities.

First degree block
- Often seen in normal people.
- Think about acute myocardial infarction and acute rheumatic fever as possible causes.
- No specific action needed.

Second degree block
- Usually indicates heart disease; often seen in acute myocardial infarction.
- Mobitz type 2 and Wenckebach block do not need specific treatment.
- 2:1 block may indicate a need for temporary or permanent pacing, especially if the ventricular rate is slow.

Third degree block
- Always indicates conducting tissue disease – more often fibrosis than ischaemic.
- Consider a temporary or permanent pacemaker.

Right bundle branch block
- Think about an atrial septal defect.
- No specific treatment.

Left bundle branch block
- Think about aortic stenosis and ischaemic disease.
- If the patient is asymptomatic, no action is needed.

- If the patient has recently had severe chest pain, LBBB may indicate an acute myocardial infarction, and thrombolysis should be considered.

Left axis deviation
- Think about left ventricular hypertrophy.
- No action needed.

Left axis deviation and right bundle branch block
- Indicates severe conducting tissue disease.
- No specific treatment needed.
- Pacemaker required if the patient has symptoms suggestive of intermittent complete heart block.

THINGS TO REMEMBER

1. Depolarization normally begins in the SA node, and spreads to the ventricles via the AV node, the His bundle, the right and left branches of the His bundle, and the anterior and posterior fascicles of the left bundle branch.
2. A conduction abnormality can develop at any of these points.
3. Conduction problems in the AV node and His bundle may be partial (first and second degree block) or complete (third degree block).
4. If conduction is normal through the AV node, the His bundle and one of its branches, but is abnormal in the other branch, bundle branch block exists and the QRS complex is wide.
5. The ECG pattern of RBBB and LBBB can be worked out if you remember (a) that the septum is depolarized first from left to right; (b) that lead V_1 looks at the right ventricle and lead V_6 at the left ventricle; and (c) that when depolarization spreads towards an electrode the stylus moves upwards.

6. If you can't remember all this, remember that RBBB has an RSR^1 pattern in lead V_1, while LBBB has a letter 'M' pattern in lead V_6.
7. Block of the anterior division or fascicle of the left bundle branch causes left axis deviation.

3
The rhythm of the heart

So far we have only considered the spread of depolarization that follows the normal activation of the sinoatrial (SA) node. When depolarization begins in the SA node the heart is said to be in sinus rhythm. Depolarization can, however, begin in other places. Then the rhythm is named after the part of the heart where the depolarization sequence originates, and an 'arrhythmia' is said to be present. Remember:

- Abnormalities of cardiac rhythm are easy to work out. The two things to look at are the P waves and the width of the QRS complexes.

When attempting to analyse a cardiac rhythm remember:

- Atrial contraction is associated with the P wave of the ECG.
- Ventricular contraction is associated with the QRS complex.
- Atrial contraction normally precedes ventricular contraction, and there is normally one atrial contraction per ventricular contraction (i.e. there should be as many P waves as there are QRS complexes).

THE INTRINSIC RHYTHMICITY OF THE HEART

Most parts of the heart can depolarize spontaneously and rhythmically, and the rate of contraction of the ventricles will be controlled by the part of the heart that is depolarizing most frequently. The SA node normally has the highest frequency of discharge. Therefore the rate of contraction of the ventricles will equal the rate of discharge of the SA node.

The rate of discharge of the SA node is influenced by the vagus nerves, and reflexes originating in the lung also affect the heart rate. Changes in heart rate associated with respiration are normally seen in young people, and this is called 'sinus arrhythmia' (Fig. 3.1).

A slow sinus rhythm ('sinus bradycardia') is associated with athletic training, fainting attacks, hypothermia and myxoedema, and it is often seen immediately after a heart attack. A fast sinus rhythm ('sinus tachycardia') is associated with exercise, fear, pain, haemorrhage and thyrotoxicosis. There is no particular rate that is called 'bradycardia' or 'tachycardia' – these are merely descriptive terms.

Abnormal cardiac rhythms can begin in three places – the atrial muscle; the region around the AV node (this rhythm is called 'nodal' or, more properly, 'junctional'); or the ventricular muscle. In Figure 3.2 the stars suggest

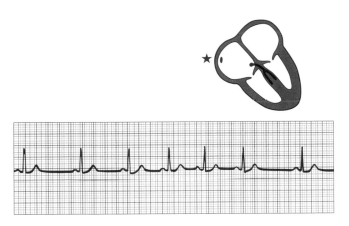

Fig. 3.1 Sinus arrhythmia

Note
- One P wave per QRS complex
- Constant PR interval
- Progressive beat-to-beat change in R-R interval

The star in this and other figures in this chapter indicates the part of the heart where the activation sequence began

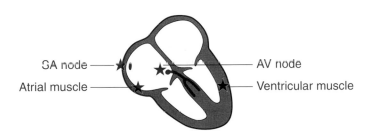

SA node ——— ★   ——— AV node
Atrial muscle ——— ★   ——— Ventricular muscle

Fig. 3.2 Points where cardiac rhythms can begin

specific points within the atrial and ventricular muscles at which electrical activation might begin, but abnormal rhythms can begin anywhere within the atrial or ventricular muscle.

Sinus rhythm, atrial rhythm, and junctional rhythm together constitute the 'supraventricular' rhythms (Fig. 3.3).

In the supraventricular rhythms, the depolarization wave spreads to the ventricles in the normal way via the His bundle and its branches (Fig. 3.4). The QRS complex is therefore normal, and is the same whether depolarization

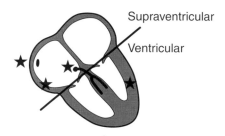

Fig. 3.3 **Division of abnormal rhythms into supraventricular and ventricular**

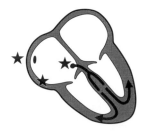

Fig. 3.4 **Spread of the depolarization wave in supraventricular rhythms**

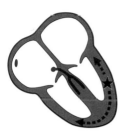

Fig. 3.5 Spread of the depolarization wave in ventricular rhythms

was initiated by the SA node, the atrial muscle, or the junctional region.

In ventricular rhythms, on the other hand, the depolarization wave spreads through the ventricles by an abnormal, and therefore slower, pathway through the Purkinje fibres (Fig. 3.5). The QRS complex is therefore wide and abnormal. Repolarization is also abnormal, so the T wave is of abnormal shape.

Remember:

1. Supraventricular rhythms have narrow QRS complexes.
2. Ventricular rhythms have wide QRS complexes.
3. The only exception to this rule occurs when there is a supraventricular rhythm with right or left bundle branch block.

TYPES OF ABNORMAL RHYTHM

Abnormal rhythms arising in the atrial muscle, the junctional region or the ventricular muscle can be slow and sustained (bradycardias); or they can occur as early single beats ('extrasystoles'); or they can be fast and sustained (tachycardias). When activation of the atria or ventricles is totally disorganized, 'fibrillation' is said to occur. We shall consider each of these types of rhythm in turn.

The escape rhythms – the bradycardias

It is clearly advantageous if different parts of the heart are able to initiate the depolarization sequence, because this gives the heart a series of 'fail-safe' mechanisms that will keep it going if the SA node fails to depolarize, or if conduction of the depolarization wave is blocked. However, the protective mechanisms must normally be inactive if competition between normal and abnormal sites of spontaneous depolarization is to be avoided. This is achieved by the secondary sites having a lower intrinsic frequency of depolarization than the SA node.

The heart is controlled by whichever site is spontaneously depolarizing most frequently: normally this is the SA node, and it gives a normal heart rate of about 70/min. If the SA node fails to depolarize, control will be assumed by a focus either in the atrial muscle or in the region around the AV node (the junctional region), both of which have spontaneous depolarization frequencies of about 50/min. If these fail, or if conduction through the His bundle is blocked, a ventricular focus will take over and give a ventricular rate of about 30/min.

These slow and protective rhythms are called escape rhythms, because they occur when secondary sites for initiating depolarization escape from their normal inhibition by the more active SA node.

Escape rhythms are not primary disorders, but are the response to problems higher in the conducting pathway. They are commonly seen in the acute phase of a heart attack, when they may be associated with sinus bradycardia. It is important not to try to suppress an escape rhythm, because without it the heart might stop altogether.

Atrial escape
If the rate of depolarization of the SA node slows down and a focus in the atrium takes over control of the heart, the rhythm is described as 'atrial escape' (Fig. 3.6). Atrial escape beats can occur singly.

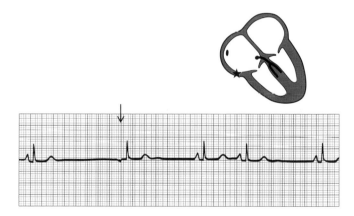

Fig. 3.6 Atrial escape

Note
• After one sinus beat the SA node fails to depolarize. After a delay, an abnormal P wave is seen because excitation of the atrium has begun somewhere away from the SA node. The abnormal P wave is followed by a normal QRS complex, because excitation has spread normally down the His bundle. The remaining beats show a return to sinus arrhythmia

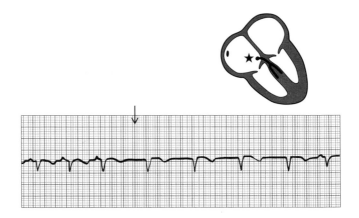

Fig. 3.7 Nodal (junctional) escape

Note

- Sinus rhythm, rate 100/min; junctional escape rhythm (following arrow), rate 70/min
- No P waves in junctional beats (indicates either no atrial contraction or P wave lost in QRS complex)
- Normal QRS complexes

Nodal (junctional) escape

If the region around the AV node takes over as the focus of depolarization, the rhythm is called 'nodal', or more properly, 'junctional' escape (Fig. 3.7).

Ventricular escape

'Ventricular escape' is most commonly seen when conduction between the atria and ventricles is interrupted by complete heart block (Fig. 3.8).

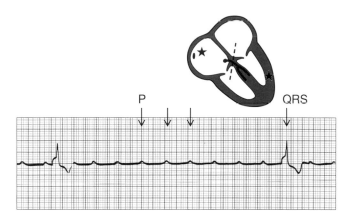

Fig. 3.8 Complete heart block

Note
- Regular P waves (normal atrial depolarization)
- P wave rate 145/min
- QRS complexes highly abnormal because of abnormal conduction through ventricular muscle
- QRS (ventricular escape) rate 15/min
- No relationship between P waves and QRS complexes

Ventricular escape rhythms can occur without complete heart block. Ventricular escape beats can be single (Fig. 3.9).

The rhythm of the heart can occasionally be controlled by a ventricular focus with an intrinsic frequency of discharge faster than that seen in complete heart block. The rhythm is called 'accelerated idioventricular rhythm' (Fig. 3.10). This is often associated with acute myocardial infarction.

Although the appearance of the ECG is similar to that of ventricular tachycardia (described later), accelerated idioventricular rhythm is benign and should not be treated. Ventricular tachycardia should not be diagnosed unless the heart rate exceeds 120/min.

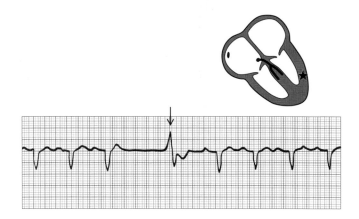

Fig. 3.9 Ventricular escape

Note
- After three sinus beats, the SA node fails to discharge. No atrial or nodal escape occurs. After a pause there is a single wide and abnormal QRS complex (arrow) with an abnormal T wave. A ventricular focus controls the heart for one beat, and sinus rhythm is then restored

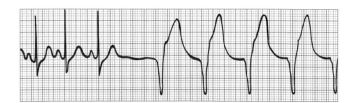

Fig. 3.10 Accelerated idioventricular rhythm

Note
- After three sinus beats, the SA node fails to depolarize. An escape focus in the ventricle takes over, causing a regular rhythm of 75/min with wide QRS complexes and abnormal T waves

EXTRASYSTOLES

Any part of the heart can depolarize earlier than it should, and the accompanying heartbeat is called an extrasystole. The term 'ectopic' is sometimes used to indicate that depolarization originated in an abnormal location, and the term 'premature contraction' means the same thing.

The ECG appearance of an extrasystole arising in either the atrial muscle, the junctional or nodal region, or the ventricular muscle, is the same as that of the corresponding escape beat – the difference is that an extrasystole comes early and an escape beat comes late.

Atrial extrasystoles have abnormal P waves (Fig. 3.11). In a junctional extrasystole either there is no P wave at all, or it appears immediately before or immediately after the QRS complex (Fig. 3.11). The QRS complexes of atrial and junctional extrasystoles are, of course, the same as those of sinus rhythm.

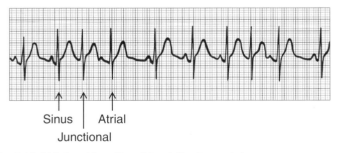

Sinus | Atrial
Junctional

Fig. 3.11 Atrial and junctional (nodal) extrasystoles

Note
- This record shows sinus rhythm with junctional and atrial extrasystoles
- A junctional extrasystole has no P wave
- An atrial extrasystole has an abnormally shaped P wave
- Sinus, junctional and atrial beats have identical QRS complexes – conduction in and beyond the bundle of His is normal

Ventricular extrasystoles, however, have abnormal QRS complexes, which are typically wide but can be of almost any shape (Fig. 3.12). Ventricular extrasystoles are common and are usually of no importance. However, when they occur early in the T wave of a preceding beat they can induce ventricular fibrillation (described later), and are thus potentially dangerous.

It may, however, not be as easy as this, particularly if a beat of supraventricular origin is conducted abnormally to the ventricles (bundle branch block, see Ch. 2). It is advisable to get into the habit of asking five questions every time an ECG is being analysed:

1. Does an early QRS complex follow an early P wave? If so, it must be an atrial extrasystole.
2. Can a P wave be seen anywhere? A junctional extrasystole may cause the appearance of a P wave very close to, and even after, the QRS complex because excitation is conducted both to the atria and to the ventricles.
3. Is the QRS complex the same shape throughout (i.e. has it the same initial direction of deflection as the normal beat, and has it the same duration)? Supraventricular beats look the same, ventricular beats look different.
4. Is the T wave the same way up as in the normal beat? In supraventricular beats, it is the same way up; in ventricular beats, it is inverted.
5. Does the next P wave after the extrasystole appear at an expected time? In both supraventricular and ventricular extrasystoles there is a ('compensatory') pause before the next heartbeat, but a supraventricular extrasystole usually upsets the normal periodicity of the SA node, so that the next SA node discharge (and P wave) comes late.

The effects of supraventricular and ventricular extrasystoles on the following P wave are as follows:

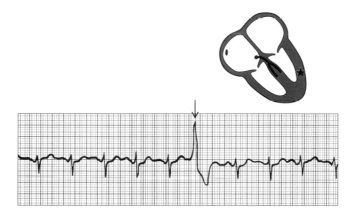

R on T phenomenon:

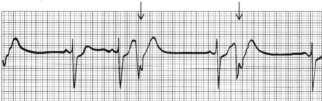

Fig. 3.12 Ventricular extrasystole

Note
- The upper trace shows five sinus beats, then an early beat with a wide QRS complex and an abnormal T wave: this is a ventricular extrasystole. In the lower trace, the ventricular extrasystoles occur (arrows) at the peak of the T waves of the preceding sinus beats: this is the 'R on T' phenomenon

- A supraventricular extrasystole resets the P wave cycle (Fig. 3.13).
- A ventricular extrasystole, on the other hand, does not affect the SA node, so the next P wave appears at the predicted time (Fig. 3.14).

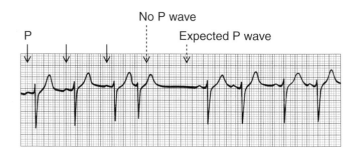

Fig. 3.13 Supraventricular extrasystole

Note

• Three sinus beats are followed by a junctional extrasystole. No P wave is seen at the expected time, and the next P wave is late

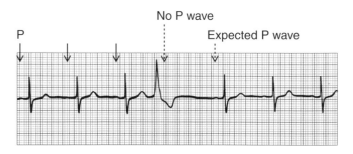

Fig. 3.14 Ventricular extrasystole

Note

• Three sinus beats are followed by a ventricular extrasystole. No P wave is seen after this beat, but the next P wave arrives on time

THE TACHYCARDIAS – THE FAST RHYTHMS

Foci in the atria, the junctional (AV nodal) region, and ventricles may depolarize repeatedly, causing a sustained tachycardia. The criteria already described can be used to decide the origin of the arrhythmia, and as before the most important thing is to try to identify a P wave.

Supraventricular tachycardias

Atrial tachycardia (abnormal focus in the atrium)
In atrial tachycardia, the atria depolarize faster than 150/min (Fig. 3.15).

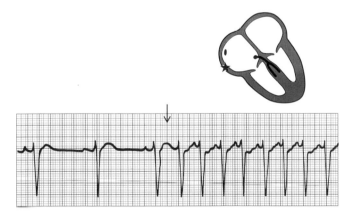

Fig. 3.15 Atrial tachycardia

Note
• After three sinus beats, atrial tachycardia develops at a rate of 150/min. P waves can be seen superimposed on the T waves of the preceding beats. The QRS complexes have the same shape as those of the sinus beats

The AV node cannot conduct atrial rates of discharge greater than about 200/min. If the atrial rate is faster than this, 'atrioventricular block' occurs, with some P waves not followed by QRS complexes. The difference between this sort of atrioventricular block and second degree heart block is that in atrioventricular block associated with a tachycardia the AV node is functioning properly – it is preventing the ventricles from being activated at a fast (and therefore inefficient) rate. In first, second or third degree block associated with sinus rhythm the AV node and/or the His bundle are not conducting normally.

Atrial flutter

When the atrial rate is greater than 250/min, and there is no flat baseline between the P waves, 'atrial flutter' is present (Fig. 3.16).

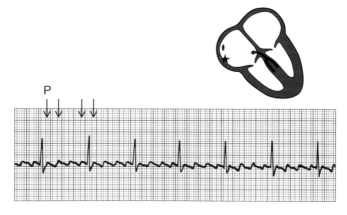

Fig. 3.16 Atrial flutter

Note
- P waves can be seen at a rate of 300/min, giving a sawtoothed appearance. There are four P waves per QRS complex, and ventricular activation is perfectly regular at 75/min

When atrial tachycardia or atrial flutter is associated with 2:1 block, you need to look carefully to recognize the extra P waves (Fig. 3.17). A narrow complex tachycardia with a ventricular rate of 250/min should always alert you to the possibility of atrial flutter with 2:1 block.

Any arrhythmia should be identified from the lead in which P waves can most easily be seen. Full 12-lead ECGs are therefore better than 'rhythm strips'. In the record in Figure 3.18, atrial flutter is most easily seen in lead II, but it is also obvious in leads VR and VF.

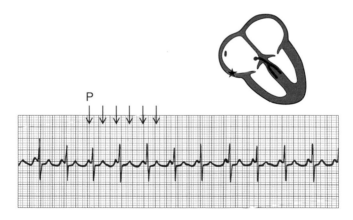

Fig. 3.17 Atrial flutter with 2:1 block

Note

- Atrial flutter with an atrial rate of 300/min is present, and there is 2:1 block, giving a ventricular rate of 150/min. The first of the two P waves associated with each QRS complex can be mistaken for the T wave of the preceding beat, but P waves can be identified by their regularity. In this trace, T waves cannot be clearly identified

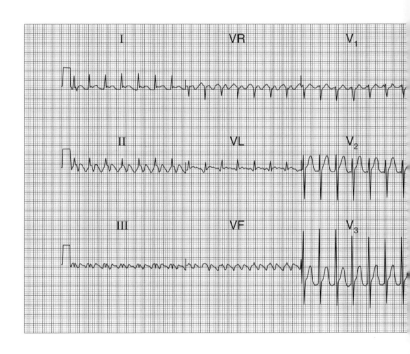

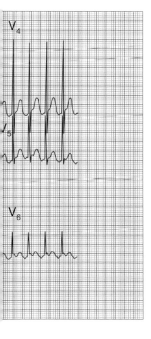

Fig. 3.18 Atrial flutter with 2:1 block

Note
- P waves at 300/min (most easily seen in leads II and VR)
- Regular QRS complexes, rate 150/min
- Narrow QRS complexes of normal shape
- Normal T waves (best seen in the V leads; in the limb leads it is difficult to distinguish between T and P waves)

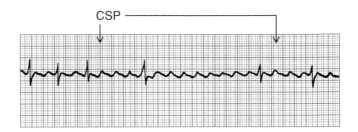

Fig. 3.19 Atrial flutter with carotid sinus pressure (CSP)

Note
- In this case, carotid sinus pressure (applied during the period indicated by the arrows) has increased the block between atria and ventricles and has made it obvious that the underlying rhythm is atrial flutter

Carotid sinus pressure may have a useful therapeutic effect on supraventricular tachycardias, and is always worth trying because it may make the nature of the arrhythmia more obvious (Fig. 3.19). Carotid sinus pressure activates a reflex that leads to vagal stimulation of the SA and AV nodes. This causes a reduction of the frequency of discharge of the SA node, and an increase in the delay of conduction in the AV node. It is the latter which is important in the diagnosis and treatment of arrhythmias. Carotid sinus pressure slows the ventricular rate in some supraventricular arrhythmias and completely abolishes others, but it has no effect on ventricular arrhythmias.

Junctional (nodal) tachycardia
If the area around the AV node depolarizes frequently, the P waves may be seen very close to the QRS complexes (as with the corresponding extrasystoles), or may not be seen at all (Fig. 3.20). The QRS complex is of normal shape because, as

with the other supraventricular arrhythmias, the ventricles are activated via the bundle of His in the normal way.

The 12-lead ECG in Figure 3.21 shows that in a junctional tachycardia no P waves can be seen in any lead.

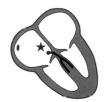

Junctional tachycardia:

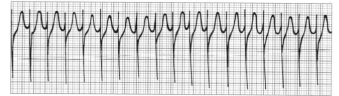

Sinus rhythm:

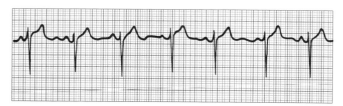

Fig. 3.20 Junctional (nodal) tachycardia

Note
- In the upper trace there are no P waves, and the QRS complexes are completely regular. The lower trace is from the same patient, in sinus rhythm. The QRS complexes have essentially the same shape as those of the junctional tachycardia

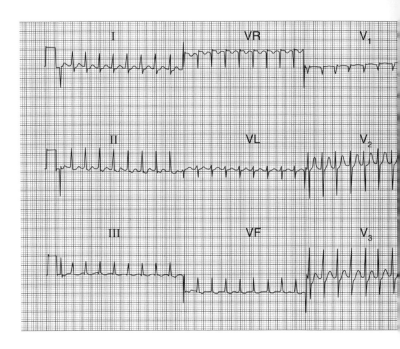

Fig. 3.22 Ventricular tachycardia

Note
- After two sinus beats, the rate increases to 150/min. The QRS complexes become broad, and the T waves are difficult to identify. The final beat shows a return to sinus rhythm

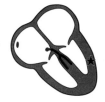

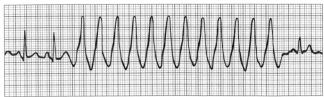

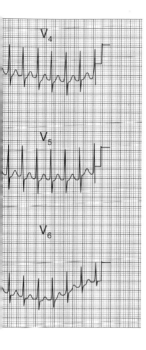

Fig. 3.21 Supraventricular tachycardia

Note
- No P waves
- Regular QRS complexes, rate 180/min
- Narrow QRS complexes of normal shape
- Normal T waves
- Treatment: carotid sinus pressure, then adenosine if necessary

Ventricular tachycardias

If a focus in the ventricular muscle depolarizes with high frequency (causing, in effect, rapidly repeated ventricular extrasystoles), the rhythm is called 'ventricular tachycardia' (Fig. 3.22). Excitation has to spread by an abnormal path through the ventricular muscle, and the QRS complex is therefore wide and abnormal.

Wide and abnormal complexes are seen in all 12 leads of the standard ECG (Fig. 3.23).

Remember that wide and abnormal complexes are also seen with bundle branch block (Fig. 3.24).

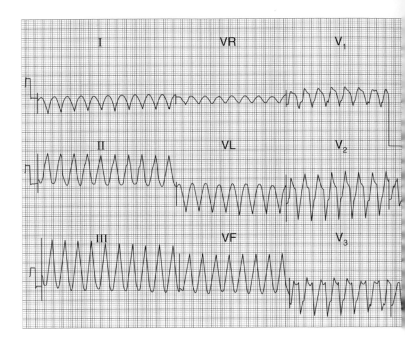

Fig. 3.24 Sinus rhythm with LBBB

Note

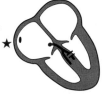

- Sinus rhythm: each QRS complex is preceded by a P wave, with a constant PR interval. The QRS complexes are wide and the T waves are inverted. This trace was recorded from lead V_6, and the M pattern and inverted T wave characteristic of LBBB are easily identifiable

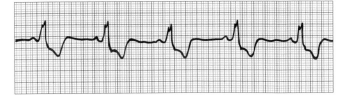

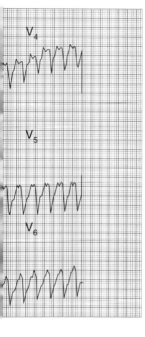

Fig. 3.23 Ventricular tachycardia

Note
- No P waves
- Regular QRS complexes, rate 200/min
- Broad QRS complexes, duration 240 ms
  with a very abnormal shape
- No identifiable T waves

How to distinguish between ventricular tachycardia and supraventricular tachycardia with bundle branch block

It is essential to remember that the patient's clinical state – whether good or bad – does not help to differentiate between the two possible causes of a tachycardia with broad QRS complexes. If a patient with an acute myocardial infarction has a broad-complex tachycardia it will almost always be a ventricular tachycardia, but a patient with episodes of such a tachycardia without an infarction could be having either a ventricular tachycardia or a supraventricular tachycardia with bundle branch block. Under such circumstances the following points may be helpful:

1. Finding P waves and seeing how they relate to the QRS complexes is always the key to identifying arrhythmias. Always look carefully at a full 12-lead ECG.
2. If possible, compare the QRS complex during the tachycardia with that during sinus rhythm. If the patient has bundle branch block when in sinus rhythm, the QRS complex during the tachycardia will have the same shape as during normal rhythm.
3. If the QRS complex is wider than four small squares (160 ms), the rhythm will probably be ventricular in origin.
4. Left axis deviation during the tachycardia usually indicates a ventricular origin, as does a change of axis compared with a record taken during sinus rhythm.
5. If during the tachycardia the QRS complex is very irregular, the rhythm is probably atrial fibrillation with bundle branch block (see below).

FIBRILLATION

All the arrhythmias discussed so far have involved the synchronous contraction of all the muscle fibres of the atria or of the ventricles, albeit at abnormal speeds. When individual muscle fibres contract independently they are said to be 'fibrillating'. Fibrillation can occur in the atrial or ventricular muscle.

When the atrial muscle fibres contract independently there are no P waves on the ECG, only an irregular line (Fig. 3.25). At times there may be flutter-like waves for 2 or 3 seconds. The AV node is continuously bombarded with depolarization waves of varying strength, and depolarization spreads at irregular intervals down the bundle of His. The AV node conducts in an 'all or none' fashion, so that the depolarization waves passing into the His bundle are of constant intensity. However, these waves

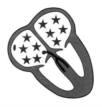

Lead II:

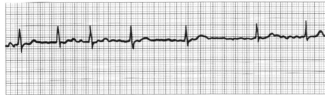

Lead V₁:

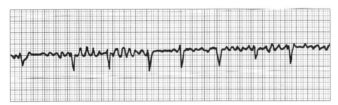

Fig. 3.25 Atrial fibrillation

Note
- No P waves – irregular baseline
- Irregular QRS complexes
- Normally shaped QRS complexes
- In lead V₁ waves can be seen with some resemblance to those seen in atrial flutter – this is common in atrial fibrillation

are irregular and the ventricles therefore contract irregularly. Because conduction into and through the ventricles is by the normal route, each QRS complex is of normal shape.

In a 12-lead record, fibrillation waves can often be seen much better in some leads than others (Fig. 3.26).

79

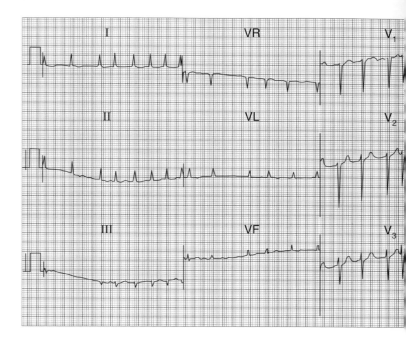

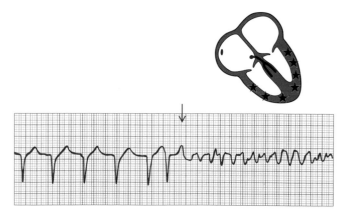

Fig. 3.27 Ventricular fibrillation

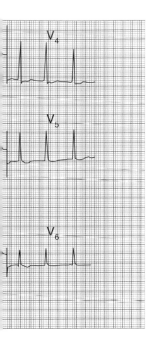

Fig. 3.26 Atrial fibrillation

Note
- No P waves
- Irregular baseline
- Irregular QRS complexes, rate varying between 80 and 180/min
- Narrow QRS complexes of normal shape
- Depressed ST segments in leads V_5–V_6
- Normal T waves

When the ventricular muscle fibres contract independently, no QRS complex can be identified and the ECG is totally disorganized (Fig. 3.27).

As the patient will usually have lost consciousness by the time you have realized that the change in the ECG pattern is not just due to a loose connection, the diagnosis is easy.

WOLFF–PARKINSON–WHITE (WPW) SYNDROME

The only normal electrical connection between the atria and ventricles is the His bundle. Some people, however, have an extra or 'accessory' conducting bundle. Accessory bundles form a direct connection between atrium and ventricle, usually on the left side of the heart, and in the

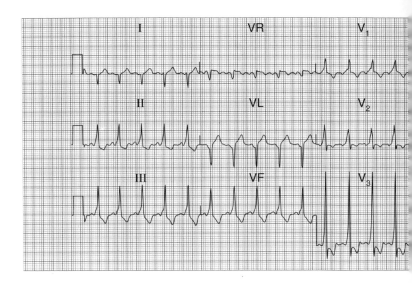

accessory bundle there is no AV node to delay conduction.
A depolarization wave therefore reaches the ventricle early
and 'pre-excitation' occurs. The PR interval is short and
the QRS complex shows an early slurred upstroke called a
'delta wave' (Fig. 3.28). The second part of the QRS complex
is normal, as conduction through the His bundle catches up
with the pre-excitation.

The only clinical importance of this anatomical
abnormality is that it can cause paroxysmal tachycardia.
Depolarization can spread down the His bundle and back
up the accessory pathway, and so reactivate the atrium. A
're-entry' circuit is thus set up, and a sustained tachycardia
occurs (Fig. 3.29).

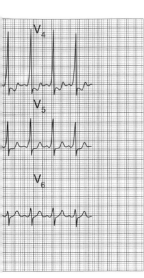

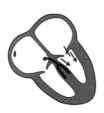

Fig. 3.28 WPW syndrome

Note
- Sinus rhythm
- Right axis
- Short PR interval
- Slurred upstroke of the QRS complex, best seen in leads V_3 and V_4. Widened QRS complex due to this 'delta' wave
- Domininant R wave in lead V_1

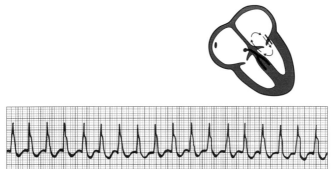

Fig. 3.29 Sustained tachycardia in the WPW syndrome

Note
- During re-entry tachycardia, no P waves can be seen

THE ORIGINS OF TACHYCARDIAS

We have considered the tachycardias up to now as if all were due to an increased spontaneous frequency of depolarization of some part of the heart. While such an 'enhanced automaticity' certainly accounts for some tachycardias, others are due to re-entry circuits within the heart muscle. It is not possible to distinguish enhanced automaticity from re-entry tachycardia on standard ECGs, but fortunately this differentiation has no practical importance.

WHAT TO DO

Accurate interpretation of the ECG is an essential part of arrhythmia management. Although this book is not intended to discuss therapy in any detail, it seems appropriate to outline some simple approaches to patient management that logically follow interpretation of an ECG recording:

1. For fast or slow sinus rhythm, treat the underlying cause, not the rhythm itself.
2. Extrasystoles rarely need treatment.
3. In patients with acute heart failure or low blood pressure due to a tachycardia, DC cardioversion should be considered early on.
4. Patients with any bradycardia that is affecting the circulation can be treated with atropine, but if this is ineffective they will need temporary or permanent pacing (Fig. 3.30).

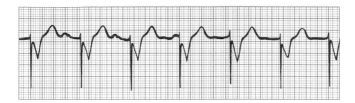

Fig. 3.30 Pacemaker

Note
- Occasional P waves are visible, but are not related to the QRS complexes. The QRS complexes are preceded by a brief spike, representing the pacemaker stimulus. The QRS complexes are broad, because pacemakers stimulate the right ventricle and cause 'ventricular' beats

5. The first treatment for any abnormal tachycardia is carotid sinus pressure. This should be performed with the ECG running, and may help make the diagnosis:
   - Sinus tachycardia – carotid sinus pressure causes temporary slowing of the heart rate
   - Atrial and junctional tachycardia – carotid sinus pressure may terminate the arrhythmia or may have no effect
   - Atrial flutter – carotid sinus pressure usually causes a temporary increase in block (e.g. from 2:1 to 3:1)
   - Atrial fibrillation and ventricular tachycardia – carotid sinus pressure has no effect.
6. Narrow complex tachycardias should be treated initially with adenosine.
7. Wide complex tachycardias should be treated initially with lignocaine.

THINGS TO REMEMBER

1. Most parts of the heart are capable of spontaneous depolarization.
2. Abnormal rhythms can arise in the atrial muscle, the region around the AV node (the junctional region) and in the ventricular muscle.
3. Escape rhythms are slow and are protective.
4. Occasional early depolarization of any part of the heart causes an extrasystole.
5. Frequent depolarization of any part of the heart causes a tachycardia.
6. Asynchronous contraction of muscle fibres in the atria or ventricles is called fibrillation.
7. Apart from the rate, the ECG pattern of an escape rhythm, an extrasystole and a tachycardia arising in any one part of the heart are the same.
8. All supraventricular rhythms have normal QRS complexes provided there is no bundle branch block (see Ch. 2).
9. Ventricular rhythms cause wide and abnormal QRS complexes, and abnormal T waves.

Recognizing ECG abnormalities is to a large extent like recognizing an elephant – once seen, never forgotten. However, in cases of difficulty it is helpful to ask the following questions, referring to Table 3.1:

1. Is the abnormality occasional or sustained?
2. Are there any P waves?
3. Are there as many QRS complexes as P waves?
4. Are the ventricles contracting regularly or irregularly?
5. Is the QRS complex of normal shape?
6. What is the ventricular rate?

Table 3.1 Recognizing ECG abnormalities

Abnormality	P wave	P:QRS ratio	QRS regularity	QRS shape	QRS rate	Rhythm
Occasional (i.e. extrasystoles)				Normal		Supraventricular
				Abnormal		Ventricular
Sustained	Present	P:QRS = l:l	Regular	Normal	Normal	Sinus rhythm
					≥ 160/min	Atrial tachycardia
			Slightly irregular	Normal	Normal	Sinus arrhythmia
					Slow	Atrial escape
		More P waves than QRS	Regular	Normal	Fast	Atrial tachycardia with block
					Slow	Second degree heart block
				Abnormal	Slow	Complete heart block
	Absent		Regular	Normal	Fast	Nodal tachycardia
					Slow	Nodal escape
				Abnormal	Fast	Nodal tachycardia with bundle branch block or ventricular tachycardia
			Slightly irregular	Abnormal	Fast	Ventricular tachycardia
			Very irregular	Normal	Any speed	Atrial fibrillation
		QRS absent				Ventricular fibrillation or standstill

4

Abnormalities of P waves, QRS complexes and T waves

When interpreting an ECG, identify the rhythm first. Then ask the following questions – always in the same sequence:

1. Are there any abnormalities of the P wave?
2. What is the cardiac axis? (Look at the QRS complex in leads I, II, III – and at Chapter 1 if necessary)
3. Is the QRS complex of normal duration?
4. Are there any other abnormalities in the QRS complex – particularly, are there any abnormal Q waves?
5. Is the ST segment raised or depressed?
6. Is the T wave normal?

Remember:

1. The P wave can only be normal, unusually tall, or unusually broad.
2. The QRS complex can only have three abnormalities – it can be too broad, too tall, and it may contain an abnormal Q wave.
3. The ST segment can only be normal, elevated or depressed.
4. The T wave can only be the right way up or the wrong way up.

ABNORMALITIES OF THE P WAVE

Apart from alterations of the shape of the P wave associated with rhythm changes, there are only two important abnormalities:

1. Anything that causes the right atrium to become hypertrophied (such as tricuspid valve stenosis or pulmonary hypertension) causes the P wave to become peaked (Fig. 4.1).
2. Left atrial hypertrophy (usually due to mitral stenosis) causes a broad and bifid P wave (Fig. 4.2).

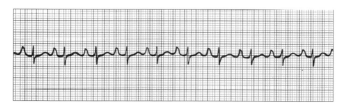

Fig. 4.1 Right atrial hypertrophy

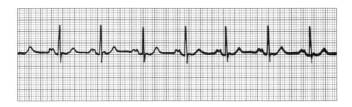

Fig. 4.2 Left atrial hypertrophy

ABNORMALITIES OF THE QRS COMPLEX

The normal QRS complex has four characteristics:

1. Its duration is no greater than 120 ms (three small squares)
2. In a right ventricular lead (V_1), the S wave is greater than the R wave
3. In a left ventricular lead (V_5 or V_6), the height of the R wave is less than 25 mm
4. Left ventricular leads may show Q waves due to septal depolarization, but these are less than 1 mm across and less than 2 mm deep.

Abnormalities of the width of the QRS complex

QRS complexes are abnormally wide in the presence of bundle branch block (see Ch. 2) or when depolarization is initiated by a focus in the ventricular muscle causing ventricular escape beats, extrasystoles or tachycardia (see Ch. 3). In either case, the increased width indicates that depolarization has spread through the ventricles by an abnormal and therefore slow pathway.

Increased height of the QRS complex

An increase of muscle mass in either ventricle will lead to increased electrical activity, and to an increase in the height

of the QRS complex.

Right ventricular hypertrophy

Right ventricular hypertrophy is best seen in the right ventricular leads (especially V_1). Since the left ventricle does not have its usual dominant effect on the QRS shape, the complex becomes upright (i.e. the height of the R wave exceeds the depth of the S wave) – this is nearly always abnormal (Fig. 4.3). There will be a deep S wave in lead V_6.

Right ventricular hypertrophy is usually accompanied by right axis deviation (see Ch. 1), by a peaked P wave (right atrial hypertrophy), and in severe cases by inversion of the T waves in leads V_1 and V_2, and sometimes in lead V_3 or even V_4 (Fig. 4.4).

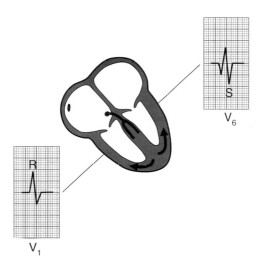

Fig. 4.3 Conduction in right ventricular hypertrophy

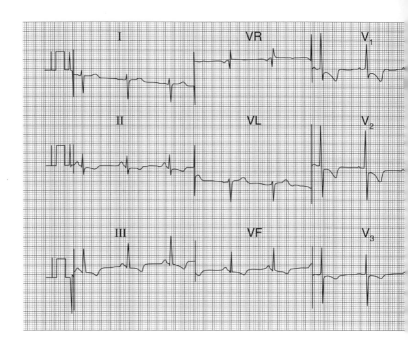

Pulmonary embolism

In pulmonary embolism the ECG may show features of
right ventricular hypertrophy, although in many cases there
is nothing abnormal other than a sinus tachycardia. When a
pulmonary embolus is suspected, look for:

1. Peaked P waves
2. Right axis deviation (S waves in lead I)
3. Tall R waves in lead V_1
4. Right bundle branch block
5. Inverted T waves in lead V_1 (normal), spreading across to
   lead V_2 or V_3
6. A shift of transition point to the left, so that the R wave
   equals the S wave in lead V_5 or V_6 rather than in lead V_3 or
   V_4 (clockwise rotation). A deep S wave will persist in lead V_6

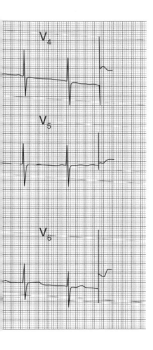

Fig. 4.4 Severe right ventricular hypertrophy

Notes
- Sinus rhythm
- Right axis deviation (deep S waves in lead I)
- Dominant R waves in lead V_1
- Deep S waves in lead V_6 (clockwise rotation)
- Inverted T waves in leads I, II, III, VF, V_1–V_4

7. Curiously, a 'Q' wave in lead III resembling an inferior infarction (see later).

However, do not hesitate to treat the patient if the clinical picture suggests pulmonary embolism but the ECG does not show the classical pattern of right ventricular hypertrophy. If in doubt, treat the patient with an anticoagulant.

Left ventricular hypertrophy
Left ventricular hypertrophy causes a tall R wave (greater than 25 mm) in lead V_5 or V_6 and a deep S wave in lead V_1 or V_2 (Fig. 4.5) – but in practice such 'voltage' changes alone are unhelpful in diagnosing left ventricular enlargement. With significant hypertrophy, there are also inverted T waves in leads I, VL, V_5 and V_6, and sometimes V_4, and there

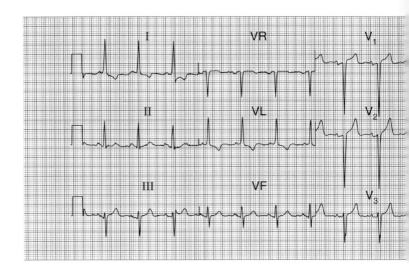

may be left axis deviation. It is difficult to diagnose minor degrees of left ventricular hypertrophy from the ECG.

The origin of Q waves

Small (septal) 'Q' waves in the left ventricular leads result from depolarization of the septum from left to right (see Ch. 1). However, Q waves greater than one small square in width (representing 40 ms), and greater than 2 mm in depth have a quite different significance.

The ventricles are depolarized from inside outwards (Fig. 4.6). Therefore, an electrode placed in the cavity of a ventricle would record only a Q wave, because all the depolarization waves would be moving away from it. If a myocardial infarction causes complete death of muscle from the inside surface to the outside surface of the heart, an electrical 'window' is created, and an electrode looking at the heart over that window will record a cavity potential – that is, a Q wave.

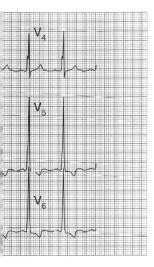

Fig. 4.5 Left ventricular hypertrophy

Notes
- Sinus rhythm
- Normal axis
- Tall R waves in leads V_5, V_6, and deep S waves in leads V_1, V_2 (R wave in lead V_1, 40 mm)
- Inverted T waves in leads I, II, V_5, V_6

Q waves greater than one small square in width and at least 2 mm deep therefore indicate a myocardial infarction, and the leads in which the Q wave appears give some indication of the part of the heart that has been damaged. Thus, infarction of the anterior wall of the left ventricle

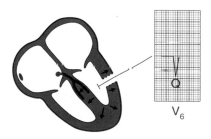

Fig. 4.6 The origin of Q waves

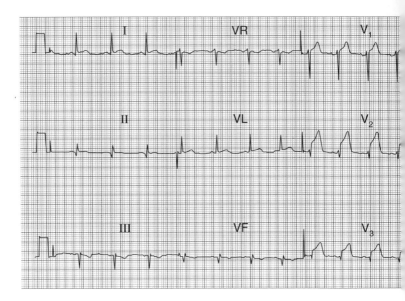

causes a Q wave in the leads looking at the heart from the front – V_2–V_4 or V_5 (see Ch. 1) (Fig. 4.7).

If the infarction involves both the anterior and lateral surfaces of the heart, a Q wave will be present in leads V_3 and V_4 and in the leads that look at the lateral surface – I, VL and V_5–V_6 (Fig. 4.8).

Infarctions of the inferior surface of the heart cause Q waves in the leads looking at the heart from below – III and VF (Figs 4.7 and 4.9).

When the posterior wall of the left ventricle is infarcted, a different pattern is seen. The right ventricle occupies the front of the heart anatomically, and normally depolarization of the right ventricle (moving towards the recording electrode V_1) is overshadowed by depolarization of the left

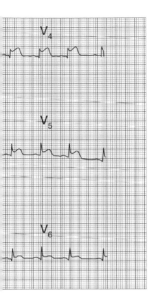

Fig. 4.7 Acute myocardial infarction, and probable old inferior infarction (see Fig. 4.13)

Notes
- Sinus rhythm with a normal rhythm
- Small Q waves in leads II, III, VF
- Raised ST segments in leads V_2–V_5
- Inverted T wave in leads III, VF

ventricle (moving away from V_1). The result is a dominant S wave in lead V_1 (see Ch. 1). With infarction of the posterior wall of the left ventricle, depolarization of the right ventricle is less opposed by left ventricular forces, and so becomes more obvious and a dominant R wave develops in lead V_1. The appearance of the ECG is similar to that of right ventricular hypertrophy, though the other changes of right ventricular hypertrophy (see above) do not appear.

The presence of a Q wave does not give any indication of the age of an infarction, because once a Q wave has developed it is usually permanent.

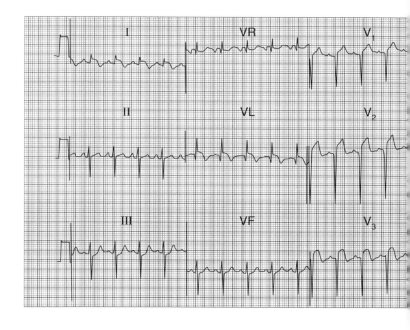

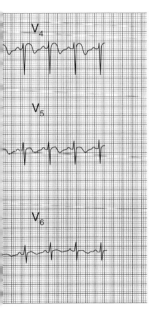

Fig. 4.8 Acute anterolateral myocardial infarction

Notes
- Sinus rhythm
- Left axis (dominant S waves in leads II and III)
- Q wave in leads VL, V_3
- Raised ST segments in leads I, VL, V_2–V_5

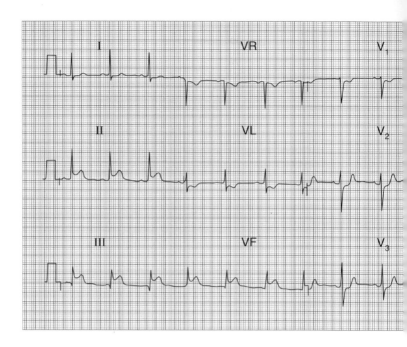

ABNORMALITIES OF THE ST SEGMENT

The ST segment lies between the QRS complex and the T wave (Fig. 4.10).

It should be 'isoelectric' – that is, at the same level as the part between the T wave and the next P wave – but it may be elevated (Fig. 4.11a) or depressed (Fig. 4.11b).

Elevation of the ST segment is an indication of acute myocardial injury, usually due either to a recent infarction or to pericarditis. The leads in which the elevation occurs indicate the part of the heart that is damaged – anterior damage shows in the V leads, and inferior damage in leads III and VF (see Figs 4.7–4.9). Pericarditis is not usually a localized affair, and so it causes ST elevation in most leads.

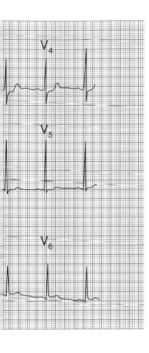

Fig. 4.9 Acute inferior infarction; lateral ischaemia

Notes
- Sinus rhythm
- Normal axis
- Normal QRS complexes
- Raised ST segments in leads II, III, VF
- Inverted T waves in lead VL and in V_1, which is normal

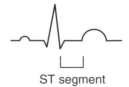

ST segment

Fig. 4.10 The ST segment

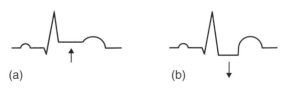

(a)   (b)

Fig. 4.11 (a) Elevated ST segment. (b) Depressed ST segment

Rest:

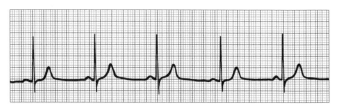

Exercise:

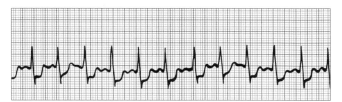

Fig. 4.12 Exercise-induced ischaemic changes

Note
- In the upper (normal) trace, the heart rate is 55/min and the ST segments are isoelectric. In the lower trace, the rate is 140/min and the ST segments are horizontally depressed

Horizontal depression of the ST segment, associated with an upright T wave, is usually a sign of ischaemia as opposed to infarction. When the ECG at rest is normal, ST segment depression may appear during exercise, particularly when effort induces angina (Fig. 4.12).

Downsloping, as opposed to horizontally depressed, ST segments are usually due to treatment with digoxin (described later).

ABNORMALITIES OF THE T WAVE

T wave inversion is seen in the following circumstances:

1. Normality
2. Ischaemia
3. Ventricular hypertrophy
4. Bundle branch block
5. Digoxin treatment.

Leads adjacent to those showing inverted T waves sometimes show 'biphasic' T waves – initially upright and then inverted.

Normality
The T wave is normally inverted in leads VR and V_1 (and in lead V_2 in young people, and also in lead V_3 in some black people).

Ischaemia
After a myocardial infarction, the first abnormality seen on the ECG is elevation of the ST segment (Fig. 4.13). Subsequently Q waves appear, and the T waves become inverted. The ST segment returns to the baseline, the whole process taking a variable time but usually within the range of 24–48 hours. T wave inversion is often permanent.

If an infarction is not full thickness and so does not cause an electrical window, there will be T wave inversion but no Q waves (Fig. 4.14). This is called a 'non-Q wave infarction' pattern. The term 'subendocardial infarction' pattern is sometimes used, but it is often not pathologically correct.

1 hour after onset of pain:

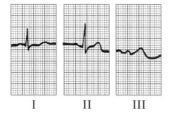

| I | II | III | VR | VL | VF |

6 hours after onset of pain:

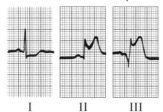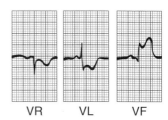

| I | II | III | VR | VL | VF |

24 hours after onset of pain:

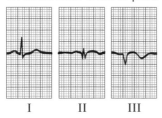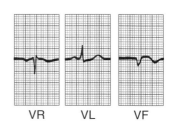

| I | II | III | VR | VL | VF |

Fig. 4.13 Development of inferior infarction

Note
- Three ECGs have been recorded over 24 hours, and have been arranged horizontally
- Sinus rhythm with a normal cardiac axis in all three ECGs
- The first record is essentially normal
- 6 hours after the onset of pain, the ST segments have risen in leads II, III and VF and the ST segment is depressed in lead VL. A Q wave has developed in lead III
- 24 hours after the onset of pain, a small Q wave has appeared in lead II and more obvious Q waves can be seen in leads III and VF. The ST segments have returned to baseline, and the T waves are now inverted in leads III and VF

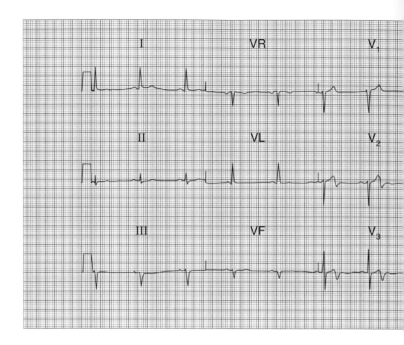

Ventricular hypertrophy

Left ventricular hypertrophy causes inverted T waves in leads looking at the left ventricle (V_5, V_6, II and VL) (see Fig. 4.5). Right ventricular hypertrophy causes T wave inversion in the leads looking at the right ventricle (T wave inversion is normal in lead V_1, but in white adults is abnormal in leads V_2 or V_3) (see Fig. 4.4).

Bundle branch block

The abnormal path of depolarization in bundle branch block is usually associated with an abnormal path of

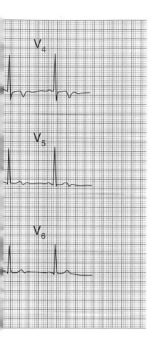

Fig. 4.14 Anterior non-Q wave infarction

Notes
- Sinus rhythm
- Normal axis
- Normal QRS complexes
- Inverted T waves in leads V_3, V_4
- Biphasic T waves in leads V_2, V_5

repolarization. Therefore, inverted T waves associated with QRS complexes which have a duration of 160 ms or more have no significance in themselves (see Figs 2.15 and 2.16).

Digoxin
The administration of digoxin causes T wave inversion, characteristically with sloping depression of the ST segment (Fig. 4.15). It is helpful to record an ECG before giving digoxin, to save later confusion about the significance of T wave changes.

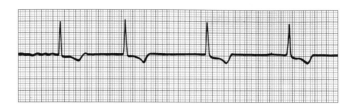

Fig. 4.15 Digoxin effect

Note
- Atrial fibrillation
- Narrow QRS complexes
- Downsloping ST segments ('reversed tick')
- Inverted T waves

OTHER ABNORMALITIES OF THE ST SEGMENT AND THE T WAVE

Electrolyte abnormalities

Abnormalities of the plasma levels of potassium, calcium and magnesium affect the ECG, though changes in the plasma sodium level do not. The T wave and QT interval (measured from the onset of the QRS complex to the end of the T wave) are most commonly affected.

A low potassium level causes T wave flattening and the appearance of a hump on the end of the T wave called a 'U' wave. A high potassium level causes peaked T waves with the disappearance of the ST segment. The QRS complex may be widened. The effects of abnormal magnesium levels are similar.

A low plasma calcium level causes prolongation of the QT interval, and a high plasma calcium level shortens it.

Non-specific changes

Minor degrees of ST segment and T wave abnormalities (T wave flattening, etc.) are usually of no great significance, and are best reported as 'non-specific ST–T changes'.

THINGS TO REMEMBER

1. Tall P waves result from right atrial hypertrophy, and broad P waves from left atrial hypertrophy.
2. Broadening of the QRS complex indicates abnormal intraventricular conduction: it is seen in bundle branch block and in complexes originating in the ventricular muscle.
3. Increased height of the QRS complex indicates ventricular hypertrophy. Right ventricular hypertrophy is seen in lead V_1, and left ventricular hypertrophy is seen in leads V_5 and V_6.
4. Q waves greater than 1 mm across and 2 mm deep indicate myocardial infarction.
5. ST segment elevation indicates acute myocardial infarction or pericarditis.
6. ST segment depression and T wave inversion may be due to ischaemia, ventricular hypertrophy, abnormal intraventricular conduction, or digoxin.
7. T wave inversion is normal in leads III, VR and V_1. T wave inversion is associated with bundle branch block, ischaemia, and ventricular hypertrophy.
8. T wave flattening or peaking with an unusually long or short QT interval may be due to electrolyte abnormalities, but many minor ST–T changes are non-specific.

And finally, remember:

- The ECG is easy to understand.
- Most abnormalities of the ECG are amenable to reason.

5
Reminders

These lists will remind you of the features that will help you recognise the patterns of normality and abnormality in the ECG.

WHAT TO LOOK FOR IN THE ECG

1. The rhythm.
2. P wave abnormalities:
   - peaked, tall – right atrial hypertrophy
   - notched, broad – left atrial hypertrophy.

3. The cardiac axis.
4. The QRS complex:
   - width:
     - if wide, ventricular origin or bundle branch block
   - height:
     - tall R waves in lead V_1 in right ventricular hypertrophy
     - tall R waves in lead V_6 in left ventricular hypertrophy
   - transition point:
     - R and S waves are equal in the chest lead over the interventricular septum, normally lead V_3 or V_4
     - clockwise rotation indicates chronic lung disease
   - Q waves.
5. The ST segment:
   - raised in acute myocardial infarction and in pericarditis
   - depressed in ischaemia and with digoxin.
6. T waves:
   - peaked in hyperkalaemia
   - flat, prolonged in hypokalaemia
   - inverted:
     - normal in some leads
     - ischaemia
     - infarction
     - left or right ventricular hypertrophy
     - pulmonary embolism
     - bundle branch block.
7. U waves:
   - can be normal
   - hypokalaemia.

THE NORMAL ECG

Limits of normal durations
- PR interval: 200 ms (5 small squares).
- QRS complex duration: 120 ms (3 small squares).
- QT interval: 400 ms (2 large squares).

Rhythm
- Sinus arrhythmia.
- Supraventricular extrasystoles are always normal.

THE CARDIAC AXIS

- Normal axis: QRS complex predominantly upward in leads I, II and III; still normal if QRS complex is downward in lead III.
- Right axis: QRS complex predominantly downward in lead I.
- Left axis: QRS complex predominantly downward in leads II and III.

Note: minor degrees of right and left axis deviation are within the normal range.

QRS complex
- Small Q waves normal in leads I, VL and V_6 (septal Q waves)
- RSR^1 pattern in lead V_1 normal if the duration is less than 120 ms (partial right bundle branch block).
- R wave smaller than S wave in lead V_1.
- R wave in lead V_6 less than 25 mm.
- R wave in lead V_6 plus S wave in lead V_1 less than 35 mm.

ST segment
- Should be isoelectric.

T wave
- May be inverted in:
  - lead III
  - lead VR
  - lead V_1
  - leads V_2 and V_3, in black people.

CONDUCTION PROBLEMS

First degree block
- One P wave per QRS complex.
- PR interval greater than 200 ms.

Second degree block
- Wenckebach: progressive PR lengthening then non-conducted P wave, and then repetition of the cycle.
- Mobitz type 2: occasional non-conducted beats.
- 2:1 (or 3:1) block: two (or three) P waves per QRS complex, with normal P wave rate.

Third degree (complete) block
- No relationship between P waves and QRS complexes.
- Usually, wide QRS complexes.
- Usual QRS complex rate less than 50/min.
- Sometimes narrow QRS complexes, rate 50–60/min.

Right bundle branch block
- QRS complex duration greater than 120 ms.
- RSR^1 pattern.
- Usually, dominant R^1 wave in lead V_1.
- Inverted T waves in lead V_1, and sometimes in leads V_2–V_3.
- Deep and wide S waves in lead V_6.

113

Left bundle branch block
- QRS complex duration greater than 120 ms.
- M pattern in lead V_6, and sometimes in leads V_4–V_5.
- No septal Q waves.
- Inverted T waves in leads I, VL, V_5–V_6 and, sometimes, V_4.

Bifascicular block
- Left anterior hemiblock (i.e. marked left axis with deep S waves in leads II and III).
- Right bundle branch block (see above).

RHYTHMS

Supraventricular rhythms
- In general:
  - narrow QRS complexes (less than 120 ms)
  - same QRS complexes as in sinus rhythm
  - normal T waves.
- Exceptions: supraventricular rhythms have wide QRS complexes with
  - bundle branch block
  - Wolff–Parkinson–White syndrome.

Ventricular rhythms
- In general:
  - wide QRS complexes (greater than 120 ms)
  - different QRS complexes from those seen in sinus rhythm
  - abnormal T waves.

Rhythm abnormalities
- Extrasystoles: single early beats suppressing the next sinus beat.
- Escape beats: absence of sinus beat followed by late single beat.

- Tachycardias.
- Bradycardias.

Common supraventricular rhythms
- Sinus rhythm.
- Atrial extrasystoles.
- Junctional (AV nodal) extrasystoles.
- Atrial tachycardia.
- Atrial flutter.
- Atrial fibrillation.
- Junctional (AV nodal) tachycardia.
- Junctional (AV nodal) escape.

Common ventricular rhythms
- Ventricular extrasystoles.
- Ventricular tachycardia.
- Ventricular escape (single beats or complete heart block).
- Ventricular fibrillation.

Supraventricular rhythms
- Sinus rhythm:
  - one P wave per QRS complex
  - P–P interval varies with respiration (sinus arrhythmia).
- Supraventricular extrasystoles:
  - early QRS complex
  - no P wave, or abnormally shaped (atrial) P wave
  - narrow and normal QRS complex
  - normal T wave
  - next P wave is 'reset'.
- Atrial tachycardia:
  - QRS complex rate greater than 150/min
  - abnormal P waves, usually with short PR intervals
  - usually one P wave per QRS complex, but sometimes P wave rate 200–240/min, with 2:1 block.

- Atrial flutter:
  - P wave rate 300/min
  - sawtoothed pattern
  - 2:1, 3:1 or 4:1 block
  - block increased by carotid sinus pressure.
- Atrial fibrillation:
  - the most irregular rhythm of all
  - QRS complex rate characteristically over 160/min without treatment, but can be slower
  - no P waves identifiable, but there is a varying, completely irregular baseline.
- Junctional (AV nodal) tachycardia:
  - commonly, but inappropriately, called 'SVT' (supraventricular tachycardia)
  - no P waves
  - rate usually 150–180/min
  - carotid sinus pressure may cause reversion to sinus rhythm.
- Escape rhythms:
  - bradycardias, otherwise characteristics as above, except that atrial fibrillation does not occur as an escape rhythm.

Ventricular rhythms

- Ventricular extrasystoles:
  - early QRS complex
  - no P wave
  - QRS complex wide (greater than 120 ms)
  - abnormally shaped QRS complex
  - abnormally shaped T wave
  - next P wave is on time.
- Ventricular tachycardia:
  - no P waves
  - QRS complex rate greater than 160/min
  - accelerated idioventricular rhythm: as for ventricular tachycardia, but QRS complex rate less than 120/min.

- Ventricular fibrillation:
  - look at the patient, not the ECG.

MYOCARDIAL INFARCTION

Sequence of ECG changes
1. Normal ECG.
2. Raised ST segments.
3. Appearance of Q waves.
4. Normalization of ST segments.
5. Inversion of T waves.

Site of infarction
- Anterior infarction: changes classically in leads V_3–V_4, but often also in leads V_2–V_5.
- Inferior infarction: changes in leads III and VF.
- Lateral infarction: changes in leads I, VL, V_5–V_6.
- True posterior infarction: dominant R waves in lead V_1.

PULMONARY EMBOLISM

Possible ECG patterns include:

- Normal ECG with sinus tachycardia.
- Peaked P waves.
- Right axis deviation.
- Right bundle branch block.
- Dominant R waves in lead V_1 (i.e. R wave bigger than S wave).
- Inverted T waves in leads V_1–V_3.
- Deep S waves in lead V_6.
- Right axis (S waves in lead I), plus Q waves and inverted T waves in lead III.

HYPERTROPHY OF THE HEART

Right ventricular hypertrophy
- Tall R waves in lead V_1.
- T wave inversion in leads V_1 and V_2, and sometimes in V_3 and even V_4.
- Deep S waves in lead V_6.
- Right axis deviation.
- Sometimes, right bundle branch block.

Left ventricular hypertrophy
- R waves in lead V_5 or V_6 greater than 25 mm.
- R waves in lead V_5 or V_6 plus S waves in lead V_1 or V_2 greater than 35 mm.
- Inverted T waves in leads I, VL, V_5–V_6 and, sometimes, V_4.

Left atrial hypertrophy
- Bifid P waves.

Right atrial hypertrophy
- Peaked P waves.

DIFFERENTIAL DIAGNOSIS OF ECG CHANGES

We can rearrange some of these lists to remind you of the possible implications of ECG patterns.

P:QRS apparently not 1:1
If you cannot see one P wave per QRS complex, consider the following:

1. P wave present but not easily visible: look particularly at leads II and V_1.
2. If QRS complexes are irregular, the rhythm is probably atrial fibrillation and what seem to be P waves actually are not.

3. If the QRS complex rate is rapid and there are no P waves, a wide QRS complex indicates ventricular tachycardia and a narrow QRS complex indicates junctional (AV nodal) tachycardia.
4. If the QRS complex rate is slow, it is probably an escape rhythm.

P:QRS more than 1:1

If you can see more P waves than QRS complexes, consider the following:

1. If the P wave rate is 300/min, the rhythm is atrial flutter.
2. If the P wave rate is 150–200/min and there are two Q waves per QRS complex, the rhythm is atrial tachycardia with block.
3. If the P wave rate is normal (e.g. 60–100/min) and there is 2:1 conduction, the rhythm is sinus with second degree block.
4. If the PR interval appears to be different with each beat, complete (third degree) heart block is probably present.

Wide QRS complexes (greater than 120 ms)

Wide QRS complexes are characteristic of:

- Sinus rhythm with bundle branch block.
- Sinus rhythm with Wolff–Parkinson–White syndrome.
- Ventricular extrasystoles.
- Ventricular tachycardia.
- Complete heart block.

Q waves

- Small (septal) Q waves are normal in leads I, VL and V_6.
- Q wave in lead III but not VF is a normal variant.
- Probably indicate infarction if present in more than one lead, longer than 40 ms in duration, and deeper than 2 mm.
- Q waves in lead III but not in VF, with right axis, may indicate pulmonary embolus.
- Leads showing Q waves indicate site of infarction.

ST segment depression
- Digoxin: ST segment slopes downwards.
- Ischaemia: flat ST depression.

T wave inversion
- Normal in leads III, VR, V_1 and V_2–V_3 in black people.
- Ventricular rhythms.
- Bundle branch block.
- Myocardial infarction.
- Right or left ventricular hypertrophy.
- Wolff–Parkinson–White syndrome.

6

Now test yourself

You should now be able to recognize the common ECG patterns, and this final chapter contains ten 12-lead records for you to interpret. When reporting an ECG, remember:

- The ECG is easy.
- A report has two parts – a description and an interpretation.
- Look at all the leads, and describe the ECG in the same order every time:
  - rhythm
  - conduction – PR interval if sinus rhythm
  - cardiac axis
  - QRS complexes:
    - duration
    - height of R and S waves
  - ST segments
  - T waves.

Remember what can be normal, especially which leads can show an inverted T wave.

Then, and only then, make a diagnosis.

The ten ECGs here are in no particular sequence, but all have been described earlier in this book. Their descriptions and interpretations are given afterwards, on p. 140.

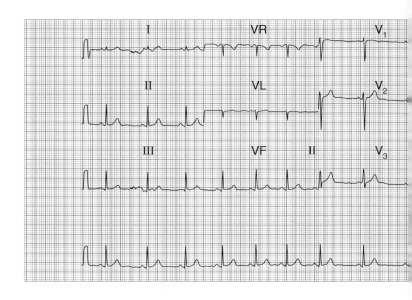

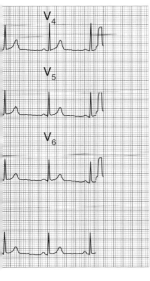

ECG 1

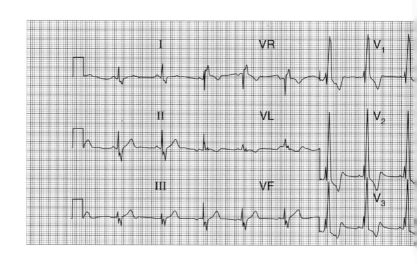

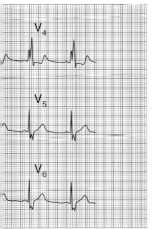

ECG 2

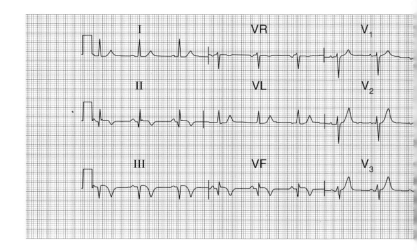

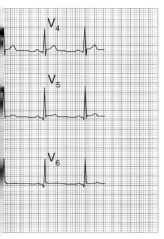

ECG 3

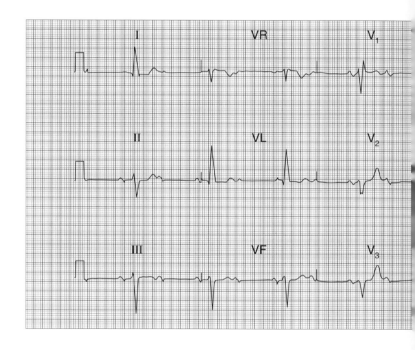

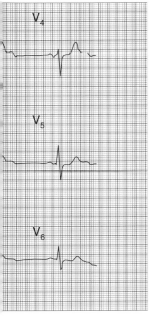

ECG 4

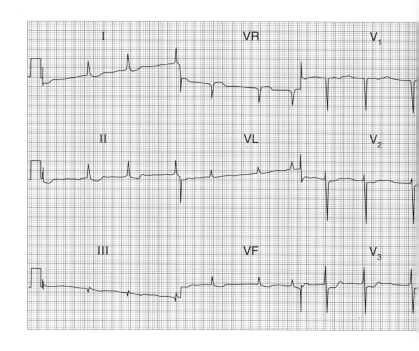

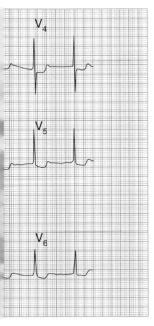

ECG 5

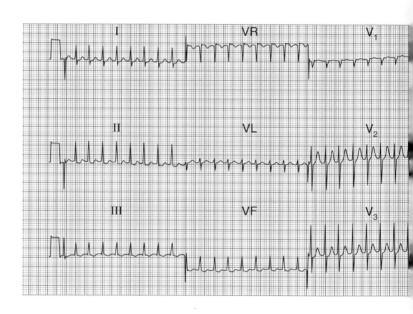

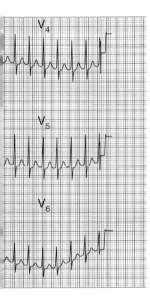

ECG 6

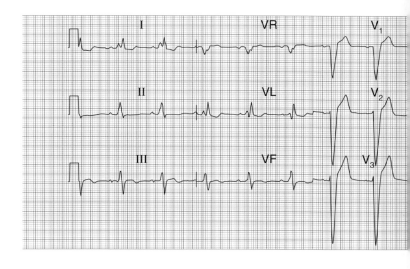

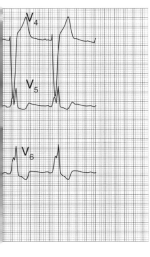

ECG 7

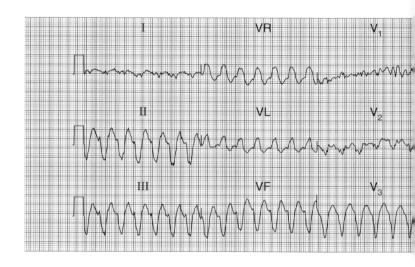

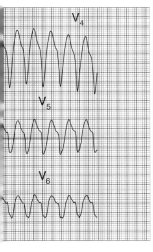

ECG 8

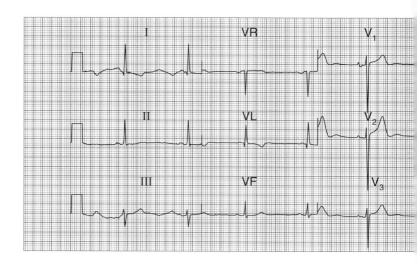

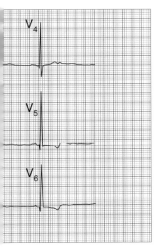

ECG 9

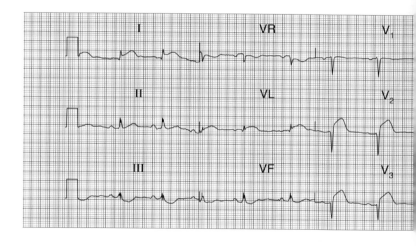

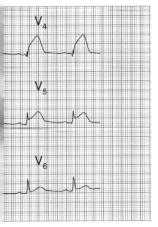

ECG 10

ECG DESCRIPTIONS AND INTERPRETATIONS

ECG 1

This ECG shows:

- Sinus rhythm; rhythm strip (lead II) shows sinus arrhythmia
- Normal PR interval 120 ms
- Normal axis
- QRS duration 80 ms, normal height
- ST segment isoelectric in all leads
- T inversion in lead VR but no other lead

Interpretation
- Normal record

If you did not get this right, look again at pages 25–27.

ECG 2

This ECG shows:

- Sinus rhythm
- Normal PR interval
- Normal axis
- Wide QRS duration, at 160 ms
- RSR pattern in lead V_1
- Wide and notched S wave in lead V_6
- ST segment isolelectric
- T inversion in leads VR (normal), V_1–V_3

Interpretation
- Right bundle branch block

Any problems? If so, look at pages 37–39 and 43.

ECG 3

This ECG shows:

- Sinus rhythm
- Normal PR interval
- Normal axis
- QRS complex – Q waves in leads II, III, VF
- ST segment isoelectric
- T waves inverted in leads II, III, VF

Interpretation
- Inferior myocardial infarction, probably old

Get this one wrong? Read pages 95–102 again.

ECG 4

This ECG shows:

- Sinus rhythm
- Alternate conducted and non-conducted beats
- Normal PR interval in the conducted beats
- Left axis deviation (deep S waves in leads II and III)
- Wide QRS complex (duration 160 ms)
- RSR[1] pattern in lead V_1

Interpretation
- Second degree (2:1) block with left anterior hemiblock and right bundle branch block, indicating severe conducting tissue disease

This was expained on page 32..

ECG 5

The ECG shows:

- Atrial fibrillation
- Normal axis
- Normal QRS complexes
- Downsloping ST segments, best seen in leads V_4–V_6
- U waves, best seen in lead V_2

Interpretation
- Atrial fibrillation of uncertain cause, with digitalis effect; U waves suggest hypokalaemia

If you made a mistake with this one, read pages 107–108.

ECG 6
This ECG shows:

- Narrow complex (i.e. QRS duration less than 120 ms) tachycardia at 200/min
- No visible P waves
- QRS complexes normal
- ST segments show a little depression in leads II, III, VF
- T waves normal except in lead III

Interpretation
- Supraventricular (junctional) tachycardia

In case of difficulty, look at pages 72–74.

ECG 7
This ECG shows:

- Sinus rhythm
- Normal PR interval
- Normal axis
- Wide QRS complex at 200 ms
- 'M' pattern in leads I, VL, V_5–V_6
- Deep S waves in leads V_4, V_5
- Downsloping ST segment in leads I, VL, V_5–V_6
- Biphasic or inverted T waves in leads I, VL V_5–V_6

Interpretation
- Left bundle branch block (remember that the deep S waves and the ST/T changes have no additional significance)

If you need to check, look at pages 39–41 and 44.

ECG 8

This ECG shows:

- Broad complex tachycardia at 160/min
- No P waves visible
- Left axis
- QRS duration 200 ms
- QRS complexes all point downwards in the chest leads (NB: lead V_1 shows artefacts)

Interpretation
- Ventricular tachycardia

The diagnosis of tachycardias is covered on pages 74–78.

ECG 9

This ECG shows

- Sinus rhythm
- Bifid P waves
- Normal conducting intervals
- Normal axis
- Tall R wave in lead V_5 and deep S wave in lead V_2
- Small (septal) Q wave in leads I, VL, V_5–V_6
- Inverted T waves in leads I, VL, V_5–V_6

Interpretation
- Left atrial and left ventricular hypertrophy

If you needed help with this one, re-read pages 90 and 93.

ECG 10

This ECG shows:

- Sinus rhythm
- Normal conducting intervals
- Normal axis
- Q wave in lead V_3
- Raised ST segments in leads I, VL, V_2–V_5
- Normal T waves

Interpretation
- Acute anterolateral myocardial infarction

You must have got this one right – the ECG is easy!

Index

Note: Page numbers in *italics* refer to figures and tables on those pages.